ALLE ZEIT WACH
1842

C. Papavasiliou Th. Cambouris
Ph. Fessas (Eds.)

Radiology of Thalassemia

With 109 Figures and 22 Tables

Springer-Verlag Berlin Heidelberg New York
London Paris Tokyo Hong Kong

Professor Dr. Constantin Papavasiliou
Department of Radiology
University of Athens, School of Medicine
Areteion Hospital
115 28 Athens, Greece

Assistant Professor Dr. Theophanis Cambouris
Department of Radiology
University of Athens, School of Medicine
Areteion Hospital
115 28 Athens, Greece

Professor Dr. Phaedon Fessas
Department of Internal Medicine
University of Athens, School of Medicine
115 28 Athens, Greece

ISBN-13:978-3-642-72589-0 e-ISBN-13:978-3-642-72587-6
DOI: 10.1007/978-3-642-72587-6

Library of Congress Cataloging-in-Publication Data
Radiology of thalassemia/C. Papvasiliou, Th. Cambouris, Ph. Fessas (eds.) p. cm. Includes index.
ISBN-13:978-3-642-72589-0 (U.S.: alk. paper)
1. Thalassemia-Diagnosis. 2. Diagnostic imaging. 3. Thalassemia-Radiotherapy. I. Papavasiliou, C. (Constantin), 1926- . II. Cambouris, Th. (Theophanis), 1930- . III. Fessas, Ph. (Phaedon) [DNLM: 1. Thalassemia-diagnosis. 2 Thalassemia-therapy. WH 170 R129] RC641.7.T5R33 1989 616.1'52-dc19
DNLM/DLC for Library of Congress 88-24976 CIP

Softcover reprint of the hardcover 1st edition 1989

2127/3145-543210 - Printed on acid-free paper

Preface

The pathophysiologic phenomena that characterize the various thalassemic syndromes result in the development of changes and lesions afflicting various tissues and organs. These changes, along with the iatrogenic ones, may be manifested by radiological means. When Cooley described the disease in 1925, for the first time, he presented the radiological bone changes, i.e., extreme osteoporosis, expansion of the diploë of the skull, retardation of bone growth, etc. Subsequent publications described radiological findings from other organs and tissues, while specialized procedures such as angiography and lymphography yielded additional information from the heart, the vessels, the lymphatics, etc.

Recent developments in ultrasonography, computerized tomography, and magnetic resonance imaging which revolutionized modern radiology have also had an impact on thalassemia, permitting a better understanding of the pathology and a more accurate evaluation of the extent and severity of the disease. This information assures proper decisions and precise selection of treatment options. Magnetic resonance imaging promises a noninvasive quantitative evaluation of the extent of active bone marrow and the degree of siderosis and probably other information as well. Nuclear medicine techniques are a valuable adjunct not only in the imaging of static pathologic processes but also in revealing and studying organ dysfunction. Although it seems paradoxical, radiation therapy has a role in the management of thalassemia, and it has been used in the management of complications caused by marrow heterotopia, a condition often associated with thalassemia. Radiation therapy in the form of total body irradiation has also been used in marrow transplantation, a method of treatment which opens new horizons in the management of these disorders. Finally, ultrasound-guided procedures contribute to prenatal diagnosis and prevention.

It is, therefore, evident that all three subspecialties of radiology, radiodiagnosis, radiotherapy, and nuclear medicine play a role in the diagnosis, evaluation, management, and prevention of thalassemia and the reader of this book may find concentrated in one volume all the relevant information.

The book is addressed to radiologists, hematologists, internists, and other physicians caring for patients suffering from thalassemia. It consists of 17 chapters and is divided into three parts. Part I deals with epidemiology, genetics, and pathophysiology. Part II is devoted to imaging, while Part III deals with management and prevention from the radiologic viewpoint.

The editors wish to thank the 22 participating authors. They acknowledge the generous help of Dr. L. M. Brown, BA, PhD, in the form of linguistic suggestions and editorial work.

They acknowledge also with gratitude permission to reproduce figures 3, 4, 5, 6, 7, 8, 10, 11 of chapter 12 from the Acta Radiologica, American Journal of Roentgenology Radiation Therapy and Nuclear Medicine, Thorax, Clinical Radiology, Journal of Computer Assisted Tomography, Radiologe and European Journal of Radiology respectively. Also the European Journal of Radiology for figures, 1, 2, 3 of chapter 13 and the Lancet for tables I and 2 of chapter 14.

A great debt of gratitude is owed to Springer-Verlag for the excellent preparation and presentation of this review.

Athens, March 1989 C. Papavasiliou

Table of Contents

Part III Management and Prevention

List of Contributors

A. Aesopos, MD
Lecturer, University of Athens, Department of Medicine, Laikon Hospital, 115 27 Athens, Greece

S. Antoniadis, MD
Pediatric Cardiologist, Hospital "Hygeia", 151 23 Athens, Greece

A. Antsaklis, MD
Assistant Professor of Obstetrics and Gynecology, University of Athens, Alexandra Hospital, 115 28 Athens, Greece

Th. Cambouris, MD
Assistant Professor, Department of Radiology, University of Athens, School of Medicine, Areteion Hospital, 115 28 Athens, Greece

I. Charib, MD
Professor of Radiology, Alexandria Faculty of Medicine, Alexandria, Egypt

A. Fertakis, MD
Associate Professor and Director, Department of Pathologic Physiology, University of Athens, School of Medicine, Laikon Hospital, 115 27 Athens, Greece

Ph. Fessas, MD
Professor and Director, Department of Internal Medicine, University of Athens, School of Medicine, 115 28 Athens, Greece

F. Franceschini, MD
Institute of Semeiotica Medica, University of Ferrara, Ferrara, Italy

A. Gouliamos, MD
Assistant Professor of Radiology, University of Athens, Department of Radiology, Areteion Hospital, 115 28 Athens, Greece

N. Gourtsoyiannis, MD
Associate Professor and Director of Radiology, University of Crete, 714 09 Hiraklion, Crete, Greece

H. Hassanein, MD
Professor of Radiology, Alexandria Faculty of Medicine, Alexandria, Egypt

D. Loukopoulos, MD
Associate Professor, First Department of Medicine, University of Athens, Medical School, Laikon Hospital, 115 27 Athens, Greece

J. Malamitsi, MD
Department of Nuclear Medicine, NIMTS Hospital, 115 21 Athens, Greece

C. Orzincolo, MD
Department of Radiology, St. Anna Hospital of Ferrara, Ferrara, Italy

A. Papaioannou, MD
Pediatric Cardiologist, Assistant Professor of Pediatrics, University of Athens, School of Medicine, 36 Voukourestiou str., 106 73 Athens, Greece

A. Papanicolaou, MD
Radiologist, Children's Hospital "Agia Sophia", 115 27 Athens, Greece

C. Papavasiliou, MD
Professor and Director, Department of Radiology, University of Athens, School of Medicine, Areteion Hospital, 115 28 Athens, Greece

J. Pappas, MD
Radiologist, IKA Hospital, 28 October 77, 153 41 Agia Paraskevi, Athens, Greece

C. Politis, MD
Director, Thalassemia Unit, Hellenic Red Cross, Athens, Greece

G. Pouliades, MD
Formerly Assistant Professor of Radiology, University of Zurich, Switzerland. Present address: 7, Dafnis str., 154 52 P. Psichiko, Athens, Greece

Y. Rombos, MD
Lecturer, University of Athens, Department of Medicine, Laikon Hospital, 115 27 Athens, Greece

P. Sfikakis, MD
Associate Professor and Director, Department of Medicine, Laikon Hospital, 115 27 Athens, Greece

D. Spigos, MD
Professor of Radiology, University of Illinois, Chairman of Radiology, Cook County Hospital, Chicago, Illin

S. Trakadas, MD
Lecturer, Department of Radiology, University of Athens,
School of Medicine, Areteion Hospital, 115 28 Athens, Greece

L. Vlahos, MD
Associate Professor of Radiology, University of Athens,
School of Medicine, Areteion Hospital, 115 28 Athens, Greece

Abbreviations

AFP	Alpha-Phyto-Proteine
AP	Anterioposterior
CA	Cooley's Anemia
CAT	Computerized Axial Tomography
CR	Conventional Radiography
CT	Computerized Tomography
CVS	Chorionic Villi Sampling
EH	Extramedullary Hemopoeisis
GVHD	Graft Versus Host Disease
Gy	Gray
Hb A	Hemoglobin A
Hb A_2	Hemoglobin A_2
Hb F	Hemoglobin F
HTR	High Transfusion Regimen
MA	Mediterranean Anemia
MH	Marrow Heterotopia
MR	Magnetic Resonance
MRI	Magnetic Resonance Imaging
MRNA	Messenger RNA
NM	Nuclear Medicine
NSD	Nominal Standard Dose
PA	Posteriointerior
PSE	Partial Splenic Embolization
RET	Roentgen Equivalent Technique
SCC	Spinal Cord Compression
TBI	Total Body Irradiation
TDF	Time Dose Fractionation
TI	Thalassemia Intermedia
Thal	Thalassemia
TM	Thalassemia Major
US	Ultrasound, Ultrasonography
YE	Yershinia Enterocolica

Part I
General

1 Introduction

Ph. Fessas

Unheard of until 1925, when Cooley and Lee under the title, "A series of cases of splenomegaly in children with anemia and peculiar bone changes", separated this syndrome from other cases of childhood anemia, thalassemia has risen gradually to an unparalleled prominence. The disease has existed with us over many millenia, if the paleo-anthropological evidence obtained from excavated skulls is being interpreted correctly.

However, migration of the abnormal genes away from their natural habitat into the healthier areas of the New World was necessary before the resulting diseases were recognized as separate morbid entities. It is reasonable to assume that in those areas in which the prevalence of thalassemia is high, it became easily confused with the many other diseases of the same zones causing splenomegaly with anemia at a young age, such as chronic malaria, leishmaniasis, congenital syphilis and perhaps severe nutritional disorders. Its designation as Mediterranean anemia, although accurate to a large extent, proved soon to be too restrictive in the geographical sense. The now prevailing name "thalassemia" does not have this shortcoming, but it is linguistically most unfortunate, especially when compared with the clear and descriptive designations of other hereditary disorders of the erythron such as spherocytosis, drepanocytosis or ovalocytosis, to name just a few. Nevertheless, it is here to stay because of continued usage, brevity and lack of a better proposal. The reader interested in the history of this group of disorders is referred to the excellent chapter of D.J. Weatherall (1980).

Although the thalassemic syndromes are caused by a very large number of mutations along the $\gamma\delta\beta$- and α-globin gene clusters (Chap. 2), which are still being mapped, data on their frequency and distribution are usually presented collectively. From the genetic and anthropological viewpoint this is obviously incorrect; as further mutations continue to be recognized, it will become necessary to be more specific when referring to geographical distribution. Additional reasons for increasing the accuracy of the genetic diagnosis are created by the feasibility of prenatal diagnosis applying DNA technology, for which exact definition of the genetic change is a prerequisite. However, from the clinical viewpoint, including all the aspects of imaging, the very refined genetic classifications may be superfluous: the clinical and hematological presentation depends much more on the degree of imbalances in globin chain synthesis created by the combination of abnormal genes and by the properties of the globin chains remaining in excess, than on the finer type of the genetic lesion. Therefore, for most clinical purposes a major distinction into α- and β-thalassemia, each group being again subdivided into mild and severe forms, may be sufficient (Chap. 3). The thalassemia zone can be pictured as a wide belt starting from the Atlantic coast of Portugal and North Africa (Morocco) and encompassing in an almost continuous fashion the populations of the northern and southern shores of the Mediterranean, including those of the Black sea, the countries of the Middle East, the population around the Caspian sea and the Persian gulf; it also covers Pakistan and the Indian subcontinent, the countries of SE Asia, notably Thailand, certain parts of southern

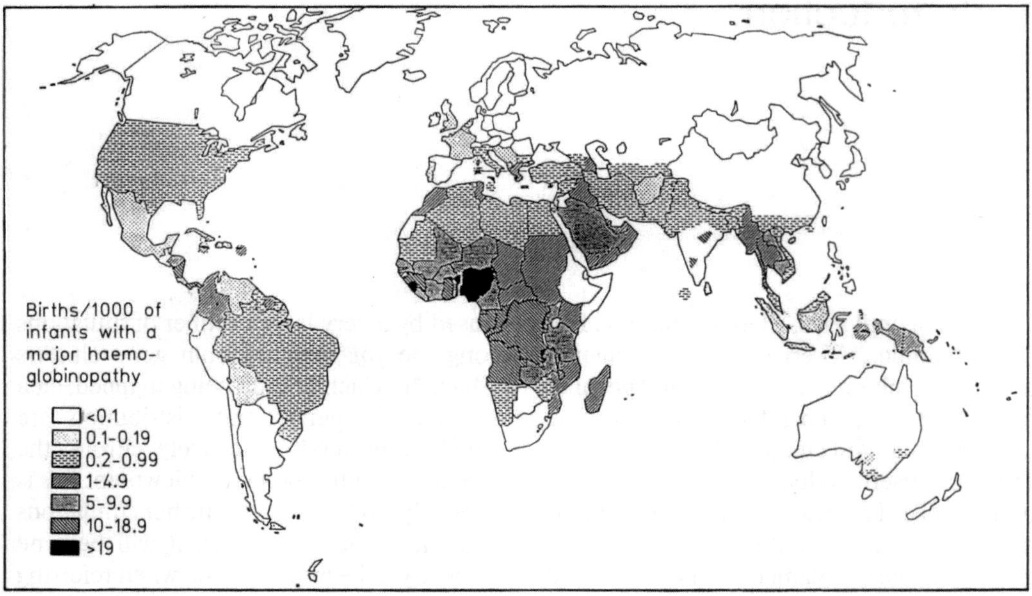

Fig. 1. World frequency distribution of major haemoglobinoparthies

China, and the archipelago of Indonesia and the Philippines, reaching New Guinea and Melanesia (Fig. 1). (Weathercall and Clegg 1981; Bunn and Forget 1986). To these areas should be added parts of the west coast of Africa. As a general rule β-thalassemia appears to predominate as compared with α-thalassemia in the western parts of the zone, which includes the Mediterranean, while as one moves eastwards the α-thalassemia varieties take precedence. Because of the interactions of *β-thalassemia* genes with structural β-chain variants, the magnitude of the problems created depends also on the presence and distribution of important abnormal hemoglobin varieties within this same belt. Thus, the β^E gene (HbE), which in association with *β-thalassemia* genes leads usually to a picture of more or less severe thalassemia intermedia, occurs in high frequences in SEAsia, Ceylon and the eastern parts of India. Also the β^Sgene (HbS, sickle cell hemoglobin) occurs in many foci on the Indian continent, the Arabian peninsula, parts of Turkey, Greece, Sicily and the southern shores of the Mediterranean; this gene interacts with *β-thalassemia* genes to cause a drepanocytic rather than a thalassemia syndrome. All other β-chain variants, numbering in the hundreds, occur in such low proportions that their possible interaction with β-thalassemia will rarely become a cause of concern. An exeption may be the variant HbO Arab, which occurs in foci around the eastern Mediterranean and Thrace and the recently reported "silent" variant Hb Knossos, identified on some Mediterranean islands, in Egypt and in Algiers, which also interacts with -thalassemia to produce thalassemia intermedia.

Along with the natural factors affecting the appearance, persistence and increase of these abnormal genes, it is evident that the map of their distribution has been determined by other conditions. Wars and conquests, slavery and forced displacement, colonization and population movements have certainly contributed over many centuries to shape the present mosaic; the entire New World and Australia have been included in the distribution of thalassemia. Even now the continuous introduction of thalassemia genes into a population relatively free of it can be seen, because of provisional or more permanent immigration to countries with a demand for workers and also because of refugees leaving the harsh conditions of their countries for better surroundings or for reasons of politics. Clearly in all these movements there is an inherent possibility for a more permanent introduction of thalassemia genes into the gene pool of populations where they were absent or very rare. Even if this does not happen, these migrant populations carry with them the medical problems connected with their genetic make-up. The medical world needs to be aware of these problems, since no area can remain immune from such gene movements.

The reason for the wide distribution and increased prevalence of thalassemia – and of the most frequent abnormal hemoglobin genes β^S, β^C and β^E – must probably be sought in a selective advantage; otherwise, the lethality of the homozygous condition, which must have been the rule in the past when no medical assistance was possible, would have led to their gradual disappearance. It is generally accepted that all these major abnormal hemoglobin genes, as well as the gene for G6PD deficiency, confer a definite protection against *Plasmodium falciparum* malaria, especially against the lethal forms which occur at younger ages. Certainly the map of distribution of falciparum malaria displays a striking similarity to the map of distribution of thalassemia genes in the Old World, and it is hard to escape the conclusion that the two phenomena are interconnected. Indeed, even a moderate degree of protection against lethal malaria in the heterozygotes, when the homozygotic condition is considered as leading to early death, may allow an abnormal gene to reach frequencies as high as 0.15 (heterozygote frequency 0.30 or 30%) within 30–40 generations.

Nowadays malaria has disappeared from many formerly infested areas. Also, thanks to better medical care – preventive and curative – it may no longer exert the severe selective pressure of former periods, even in areas where it has not been eradicated entirely. Therefore, a slow tendency to diminution of the frequencies can be exepted; this will take many generations. The trend may be offset partially by the measures of prevention applied currently through prenatal diagnosis, as well as by the better medical care permitting homozygotes to live longer and to found families.

Along with the great expansion of knowledge concerning the fundamental aspects of these syndromes, such as formal and molecular genetics, pathophysiology and molecular biology and the questions posed by related phenomena such as the switch from HbF to HbA synthesis, the reversal of this switch in thalassemia, the regulation of the balance of hemoglobin synthesis and many others which have been the result of the efforts to understand thalassemia, there has been a parallel activity in improving the management of patients (Modell and Berdoukas 1981). Within a few decades a remarkable change in the therapeutic approach towards the severe forms of the disease has occurred: from an attitude of relative, if not total, helplessness or even neglect, we have gradually progressed to the occasional transfusion, sufficient to keep the patient alive, and then to regular and more vigourous transfusion regimens, including the so-called supertransfusion or transfusion of young erythrocytes (neocytes). With such measures the growth and development of some patients has become almost normal, and this has been a very positive gain (De Sanctis 1986). However, the price paid for these satisfactory effects is also high, i.e. transfusional siderosis, of varying severity according to the success with which iron chelation can be applied. The patients stay alive, but acquire problems of a different nature, which are intensified with progressing age. Since the approaches to treating these patients have changed repeatedly within the past three decades or so, i.e. within the lifetime of many patients, it is obvious that it is difficult to accumulate sufficient numbers of matched patients who have undergone uniform schedules of therapy. If the great variability of the severity of the condition is added to the non-uniformity of therapy, a huge variety of clinical presentations is obtained, which may baffle the clinicians. Furthermore, transfusions have their own risks and complications, apart from the obligatory iron overload, especially in countries where the hepatitis B virus is also prevalent, and this happens to be true for areas with high thalassemia frequencies. To this risk should be added the newest one, transmission of HIV (human immunodeficiency virus), which will create new features in the clinical presentation of the thalassemias (Sirchia and Zanella 1987). It is the need to undergo a life-long, intense and complex therapeutic schedule, cumbersome and not totally efficient, which has been the driving force behind developments of the recent years along two major lines: the prevention of the birth of severely affected individuals by means of prenatal diagnosis and abortion, and phenotypic, therapy, through bone marrow transplantation. Thus the options for dealing with the thalassemic disorders have augmented impressively, and there is continous progress in improving both approaches by making them safer and hence more acceptable. Along with these tremendous advances there is further work to effect successful chelation of iron by means of drugs taken orally, in itself a big step to improve the patients quality of life. In a somewhat more distant future one may also hope that the realization of gene therapy will be possible (Bank et al. 1985). Meanwhile, there are sufficient concrete data indicating that manipulations of the A to F switch through pharmaceutical agents is possible to some extent; these agents are cytotoxic, but hopefully less harmful ones will be developed once the phenomena are better understood.

It is estimated that there are 200 million heterozygous carriers of abnormal hemoglobins genes worldwide; there are now many tens of thousands of severely affected patients all over the world, and close to 50 thousand new sufferers are born each year. Only a small fraction of these unfortunate individuals has the full benefit of the progress achieved in disease management, and the impact of the effective prevention will not be felt in several developing areas until many years have passed. Therefore, the thalassemia syndromes will be with us for a very long time to come. In the famework of good care and follow-up of patients, the application of imaging techniques has a very important place. Its significance increases when the patients are kept alive for many decades. The need for continuous follow-up of the chronically ill gives precedence to those imaging techniques which can be applied repeatedly without exposing the patient to undue risks, to invasive procedures or to too much incovenience. It is with this purpose in mind that this book was begun. It is the first of this kind; it is hoped that it will be useful for all who have to care for patients with thalassemia and attend to their problems. It also includes all modern approaches in the matter of prevention, namely prenatal diagnosis.

References

1. Bank A, Anderson WF, Zaino EC (eds) (1985) Fifth Cooley's anemia symposium. Ann NY Acad Sci 445
2. Bunn HF, Forget BG (1986) Hemoglobin: molecular, genetic and clinical aspects. Saunders, Philadelphia
3. De Sanctis V (ed) (1986) La maturazione sessuale nella β-talassemia major. International Meeting. Accademia delle szienze di Ferrara, suppl. vol. 63
4. Modell B, Berdoukas V (1981) The clinical approach to thalassemia. Grune and Stratton, New York
5. Sirchia G, Zanella A (eds) (1987) Thalassemia today: the Mediterranean experience. Centro transfusionale Ospedale Maggiore Policlinicio di Milano
6. Weatherall DJ (1980) Towards an understanding of the molecular biology of some common inherited anemias: the story of thalassemia. In: Wintrobe MM (ed) Blood, pure and eloquent. McGraw Hill, New York
7. Weatherall DJ, Clegg JB (1981) The thalassemia syndromes, 3d ed. Blackwell Scientific

2 Thalassemia: Basic Genetics and Molecular Defects

D. Loukopoulos

Normal Hemoglobin Synthesis

A normal red cell carries 30 pg of hemoglobin (Hb) most of which has been synthesized during the maturation of the cell in the bone marrow. Hb molecules consist of two pairs of polypeptide chains, each of which constitutes an array of 140–145 amino acids, which are assembled in an extremely precise sequence. This primary structure defines various types of chains and is of utmost importance for accurate coiling (secondary structure) and folding (tertiary structure) of the globin chain and appropriate positioning of the heme ring in its pocket. Association of two pairs of two types of chains (quartenary structure) also follows strict physicochemical rules and is crucial for the normal function of the Hb molecule.

Chain synthesis is directed by the respective genes, which are found along the DNA sequence on chromosomes 11 and 16. Like many other genes, globin chain genes are discontinuous; that is, they consist of coding and noncoding (intervening) sequences (termed exons and introns or IVS respectively), all of which are transcribed in the heterogeneous nuclear messenger RNA (hnRNA). The latter is then processed during its passage from the nucleus to the cytoplasm, where, in the form of mature mRNA, it binds to the polyribosomes and directs the synthesis of its particular chain. hnRNA processing consists of (a) capping of the 5' terminal base of the transcribed mRNA by addition of a guanine, which is subsequently methylated; (b) addition of a polyadenylic acid chain at the 3' end, which increases the stability of the mRNA during its passage from the nucleus to the cytoplasm; and (c) splicing, i.e., excision of the IVS and joining of the exons in a continous coding array.

Splicing is carried out by highly specific ribonucleases, which recognize the appropriate nucleotides at the 3' end of the coding sequences (also termed donor sites), as well as other specific nucleotide arrays prior to the 5' end of the next coding sequence (acceptor sites); cut off the intervening sequence; and join the two ends again to form the mature, continuous mRNA.

There are various forms of globin genes, which are identified by letters of the Greek alphabet. Those located on chromosome 16 constitute the α-globin gene cluster and comprise two ζ- and two α-genes. The other group (non-α-genes) is located on chromosome 11 and comprises one ε-gene, two γ-genes, one δ-gene and one β-gene. Pseudogenes, which are found among the above genes, constitute inactive sequences which resemble the active ones but have ceased to be or have never been functional. Other sequences which have a regulatory function can also be identified among the above structural genes.

The globin genes do not all function together. Instead, they are activated sequentially during ontogeny through regulatory mechanisms, most of which remain unclear as yet. This sequential activation results in synthesis of various types of chains, each of which corresponds to a specific stage of development. More specifically, during the first weeks of intrauterine life, only the ζ-genes on chromosome 16 and the ε-genes on chromosome 11 are functional; α-genes on chromosome 16 are also turned on very early. The resulting polypeptide ε, ζ-, and α-chains form the embryonic hemoglobins (Hb Gower I and II, $\zeta_2\varepsilon_2$ and $\alpha_2\varepsilon_2$ respectively). Subsequently, sequential activation of the γ-, δ-, and β-genes on chromosome 11 results in synthesis of Hb Portland ($\zeta_2\gamma_2$) in very early fetal life; fetal Hb (HbF, $\alpha_2\gamma_2$), which predominates throughout fetal life and declines rapidly after birth; and adult Hb (HbA, $\alpha_2\beta_2$), the synthesis of which also starts early in fetal life but which becomes predominant after birth. In fact, the erythrocytes of the human adult contain almost exclusively this latter pigment (98%), the rest being HbA2 ($\alpha_2\delta_2$, 2%) a minor A resulting from a late, low-rate activation of the δ-genes and, possibly, traces of HbF. The transition from HbF to HbA synthesis (switch) is a most interesting model in molecular biology because it may be retarded in certain genetic situations or be reversed under specific experimental conditions. These topics have been repeatedly reviewed in the relevant literature [1–3].

The above outline serves to make clear that normal red cell Hb synthesis is a complex procedure, the main prerequisites of which are normal structure and normal function of the globin genes. Alterations of these properties result in various forms of defective red cell Hb synthesis, which are very frequently associated with an abnormal clinical picture. As a rule, these disorders are genetically transmitted because the underlying defects are located within or very close to the affected genes. In this sense, abnormal genes are alleles of the homonymous normal ones; i.e., they occupy exactly the same positions on the homologous chromosomes and are mutually exclusive.

Inherited Abnormalities of Hb Synthesis

The above disorders are subdivided into three main groups: the hemoglobinopathies, in which one or more globin chains have an altered primary structure; the thalassemias, where the defect is expressed by reduced synthesis of one or more globin chains; and the thalassemic hemoglobinopathies, where an alteration of the primary structure of a chain also results in a decreased rate of synthesis.

According to formal genetics, an inherited Hb disorder may be heterozygous, when only one of the two allelic genes is affected, or homozygous, when both allelic genes carry the same defect. When the defect of each allele is different, the condition is defined as compound heterozygosity. Globin genes are codominant, which means that both of them are expressed, be they normal or abnormal. The resulting phenotype is determined by the nature of the defect.

Hemoglobinopathies

The majority of structural variants differ from the normal in a single amino acid residue. This change reflects a mutation of the genomic codon which substitutes a new amino acid for the normal one in the process of chain synthesis. The usual genomic defect is a base substitution. In rarer instances, the defect involves base deletions or insertions, which alter the reading frame; gene fusions, which also reduce the rate of synthesis; and base mutations at two different codons, which result in variants with two abnormal amino acid residues.

In most instances, the variant globin chain does not influence the overall function of the Hb molecule and cannot be recognized unless the amino acid substitution produces a charge difference, which allows its identification by conventional protein studies. However, in other instances, the one amino acid substitution may cause serious trouble. This topic has been extensively reviewed in the literature [4, 5] and will not be dealt with in the present chapter, except for the few frequent variants which are known to interact with the β-thalassemias and produce interesting cases of compound heterozygotes. HbS, a β-chain variant where a valine residue substitutes for glutamic acid at position 6, is a typical example of these: on releasing oxygen, $\alpha_2{}^A\beta_2{}^S$ molecules aggregate to form long bundles which transform the erythrocyte into a sickle cell, resulting in the well-known features of sickle cell diseases. The event occurs only when the intracellular concentration of HbS is high; hence, it is not produced in vivo in the heterozygous cases, where at least half of the corpuscular Hb is contributed by the normal allele. HbS occurs with high frequency in blacks and is also encountered in the Mediterranean countries and in the Indian subcontinent, where thalassemia is also a common genetic character.

Thalassemias

The term "thalassemia" now encompasses all genetic conditions where the production of one (or more) globin chain genes is subnormal or nil. The term was initially employed to denote cases with severe anemia and other typical features in children originating from countries around the Mediterranean sea [6]. Literally, it is not appropriate since it means "sea in the blood" *(thalassa* in Greek).

The thalassemias are a quite heterogeneous group. Their broad classification starts with the type of chains which are synthesized at a subnormal rate, hence the definition as α-, β-, γ, etc. thalassemias. Then, the addition of "+" or "o" denotes respectively whether the affected gene(s) function subnormally or do not function at all. In the past, further classification was based on the variety of clinical, hematologic, and biochemical features of the extremely heterogeneous patient population [7]. An indication of these groups is given in Tables 1 and 2. Today, classification of the thalassemias is based on the underlying molecular mechanisms, which in most instances can also explain satisfactorily all levels of findings.

A complete description of the molecular defects which entail reduced synthesis of a globin chain is well beyond the goals of this chapter. In summary, a gene may stop functioning when: (a) It is no longer there: Such cases occurred in the remote past by unequal crossing-over during meiotic recombination and have since been transmitted genetically to the descendants. The deletions may involve a group, one complete gene, or only a part of a gene; the result is always a zero-thalassemia. (b) The transcribed mRNA contains a premature termination signal because of a mutation along its coding sequence; the result is again a zero-thalassemia. The incomplete polypeptide chain is rapidly proteolyzed.

On the other hand, the efficiency of a gene may be decreased following a series of mutations, which (a) disturb the promotor sequences prior to the gene; (b) produce abnormal splicing of the IVS, the severity of which varies extremely from type to type; and (c) interfere with the addition of the polyadenylic acid tail, which results in a relatively unstable mRNA. As the common character of these cases is a decreased amount of normal mRNA, the respective synthesized chains are lower thal normal but not nil. These thalassemias are therefore defined as plus-thalassemias.

Another interesting group of thalassemias are due to a fusion of genes. This is again the result of an unequal crossing–over, which makes up a new gene by removing the end part of gene, the intergenic sequence, and the 5' part of another gene further downstream and joining together what is left. As a rule, the fusion genes produce the hybrid chains at a lower rate. The resulting thalassemias are considered as zero-thalassemias, with regards to the missing normal globin chains.

Last comes the group of thalassemias where the mutation transfers the termination codon further down the DNA sequence, resulting in elongated chains which are synthesized at a clearly diminished rate.

For the purposes of this book, the descriptions further below will deal mainly with the β-thalassemias. These conditions occur with high frequencies in all populations around the Mediterranean sea (Greece, Italy, North Africa, Cyprus, and the Near East) an expand, also with considerable frequencies, into the Southern Republics of the USSR, Turkey, the Middle East countries, the Indian Subcontinent [8], and Southeast Asia.

Table 1. Hematologic and biochemical parameters of the common β-thalassemia heterozygotes

Designation	Diagnostic features						Molecular defect
	Hematologic			Biochemical		Biosynthetic	
(present/former)	MCH	MCV	RBC morphology	HbA_2	HbF	β/α ratio	
β-Thalassemia Type I; high HbA_2	↓	↓	Altered (+)	↑	(↑)	< 0.5	β^0- or β^+-thalassemia due to gene deletion (partial), premature termination of the translation, or hnRNA processing abnormalties
$\delta\beta$-Thalassemia Type II; high HbF	↓	↓	(+)	↓/nl	↑	< 0.5	Deletion of both δ-β-genes; reactivation of γ-chain synthesis
Fusion $\delta\beta$-thalassemia Hb Lepore; Hb Pylos	↓	↓	(+)	↓/nl "hybrid" chains	(↑)	< 0.5	Loss of the 3' part of the β-genes and an equally long part of the 5' part of the β-gene; fusion of the remaining 5' δ and 3' β parts in a "hybrid" gene
$\gamma\delta\beta$-Thalassemia	↓	↓	(+)	↓/nl	< 0.5		Deletion of the γ-genes (no HbF), of the δ-genes (no HbA_2), and of the β-genes (low cellular HbA)

MCH, mean corpuscular hemoglobin; MCV, mean corpuscular volume; RBC, red blood cell; nl; normal key: ↓, reduced; ↑, increased; (↑), may be increased; (+), abnormal

β-Thalassemias

As a rule, heterozygous β-thalassemia is not associated with any clinical problems since the subnormal function of the defective gene(s) is adequately compensated by their normal alleles. In most cases, heterozygous carriers can be identified on the basis of the diminished mean corpuscular Hb of their red cells and by a series of more specific laboratory tests [9] (Table 1). The offspring of a carrier mating with a normal partner has a 50% probability of being homozygous normal and another 50% probability of being a carrier.

The offspring of a couple where both partners carry a β-thalassemia gene has a 25% probability of being homozygous normal, a 50% probabitily of carrying one of the two parental thalassemic genes, and a 25% probability of carrying both of them. In the latter case, a double-dose (but not always strictly homozygous) thalassemia corresponds to what is usually called thalassemia major. The clinical severity of the phenotype does not always reflect the underlying genotype. This is due to interference of various other, mostly genetic, factors, which can modify the intracellular chain imbalance and improve cellular hemoglobinization. This information is summarized in Table 2 and will be discussed

Table 2. Main features of the common phenotypes of thalassemia major in relation to the underlying molecular defects

	Clinical picture	Main laboratory findings
$\beta^{\circ}/\beta^{\circ}$-Thalassemia β°/β^{+}-Thalassemia	Severe, usually transfusion dependent	Anemia; marked RBC alterations. Reduced HbA, variable but low HbF per cell. Inclusion bodies. Normal/high HbA_2
β^{+}/β^{+}-Thalassemia	My be milder if β-chain synthesis is not greatly reduced	Mild anemia occasionally. Increased HbA, low HbF per cell. Inclusion bodies. Normal/high HbA_2
β° or $\beta^{+}/\delta\beta$-thalassemia β° or β^{+}/Fusion $\delta\beta$-thalassemia	Usually milder than the above, however, transfusion dependent in most instances	Anemia, marked RBC alterations; RBC contain inclusion bodies. Low HbA, high HbF (and "hybrid" chains), low HbA_2
$\delta\beta/\delta\beta$-Thalassemia	Usually mild (thalassemia intermedia)	Extremely mild anemia, mild RBC alterations. Red cells contain exclusively HbF (no HbA, no HbA_2), and $\delta\beta$-chains in case of fusion $\delta\beta$-thalassemia
β° or $\beta^{+}/\gamma\delta\beta$-Thalassemia	Extremely rare, severe, usually transfusion dependent	Anemia, marked RBC alterations. Reduced HbA and HbF per cell

RBC, red blood cell

in detail in the next chapter. It is noteworthy that the simultaneous presence of one or more α-thalassemia genes may occur independently and is expected to cause decreased synthesis of α-chains, which may then prove beneficial to the patient for reasons reviewed in the next section (Fertakis, Ch. 3).

Of interest in the genetics of the inherited Hb disorders is the compound heterozygosity of β-thalassemia with a β-hemoglobinopathy. In this case, the contribution of the thalassemic gene in the overall red cell Hb synthesis is minimal or nil (hence, very little or no HbA on electrophoresis); at the same time, synthesis of the variant gene continues independently and fills the red cell with the variant pigment (clearly more than the expected 50%). The condition therefore becomes quasi-homozygous for the variant, and the phenotype displays all its features, including the noxious ones.

Compound β-thalassemia/HbS heterozygotes are a typical example because their clinical picture differs little from that of homozygous sicklers. As in the thalassemias, the genotype cannot always predict the severity of the phenotype because here also other genetic modifying factors come into play. Other clinically interesting examples of compound heterozygosity are the interactions of β-thalassemia with HbE and Hb Knossos, where the phenotypes display an extremely low mean cellular Hb content because the rate of synthesis of the variant chain is also diminished [10, 11].

α-Thalassemias

The genetics of the α-thalassemias are more complex because the number of genes which can be affected is two on each chromosome. Here again the molecular mechanisms underlying the defect are deletions of one or more α-chain genes (hence, no α-chain production) or mutations leading to subnormal chain synthesis. The potential combinations are numerous and can be found in the appropriate reviews [1-3]. What is clinically important for the present introduction is the case where the total α-chain production equals approximately one-fourth of the expected total synthesis. The resulting phenotype is a mild hemolytic anemia, also known as HbH disease, the pathophysiology of which will be discussed in the next chapter. HbH disease may result from the following combinations: (a) deletion of both α-genes on one chromosome and (complete or partial) deletion of only one α-gene on the other, (b) deletion of both α-genes on one chromosome and low rate of synthesis of α-chains on the other (processing defects or elongated chains), and (c) severely reduced synthesis of α-chains on both chromosomes

References

1. Weatherall DJ, Clegg JB (1981) The thalassaemia syndromes. 3rd edn. Blackwell, Oxford
2. Nienhuis A, Anagnou NP, Ley TJ (1984) Advances in thalassemia; a review. Blood 63: 738
3. Antonarakis A, Kazazian HHJr, Orkin SH (1985) DNA polymorphisms and molecular pathology of the human globin gene clusters. Human Genet 69: 1
4. Serjeant JR, Sommeraux AM, Stevenson M et al. (1979) Comparison of sickle β-thalassemia with homozygous sickle cell disease. Br J Haematol 41: 83
5. Wintrobe MM, Lee CR, Boggs DR, Bithell TC, Athens JW, Foerster J (1981) Clinical Hematology, 8th edn. Lea and Febiger, Philadelphia
6. Whipple GH, Bradford WL (1936) Mediterranean disease thalassemia. J Pediatr 9: 289
7. Fessas Ph, Loukopoulos D (1974) The β-thalassaemias. Clin Haematol 3: 411
8. Winter WP (ed) (1986) Hemoglobin variants in human populations, vol I, II. CRC, Boca Raton
9. WHO Working Group on Community Control of Hereditary anaemias. (1982)WHO Bull 60: 643
10. Fairbanks VF, Gilchrist GS, Brimhall B, Jereb JA, Goldston EC (1979) Hemoglobin E trait reexamined; a cause of microcytosis and erythrocytosis. Blood 53: 109
11. Fessas PH, Loukopoulos D, Kokkinou S, Papasotiriou S, Karaklis A (1986) Hemoglobin Knossos: a clinical, laboratory and epidemiological study. Am J Hematol 21: 119

3 Thalassemia: Pathophysiology, Clinical and Laboratory Findings

A. Fertakis

Introduction

Thalassemias are a heterogeneous group of disorders of hemoglobin (Hb) synthesis, which have in common a reduced rate of synthesis of one or more of the globin chains of normal human Hb [25]. This leads to a variable degree of premature cell destruction, ineffective erythropoiesis and/or hemolysis, and, finally, a variable degree of anemia.

Thalassemias can be divided into two main groups, α- and β-thalassemia, depending on whether the defect in globin chain synthesis lies on the α- or β-chain respectively. Other genetic variants of thalassemia are the $\beta\delta$, δ, and $\gamma\beta\delta$ forms, in which there is a defect in the synthesis of the corresponding chain (or chains) [25].

Thalassemias are also classified according to the severity of the clinical manifestations into thalassemia major, thalassemia intermedia, thalassemia minor, and asymptomatic forms (heterozygous trait carriers).

Pathophysiology

β-Thalassemia

Despite the diversity of the different genetic forms of homozygous β-thalassemia, the clinical findings and pathophysiology are fairly similar, and these forms can be considered together. Normally, α- and β-chains are produced in almost equal quantities to form Hb A. The fundamental defect in β-thalassemia is the reduction or absence of β-chain production, as shown by a number of genetic, biochemical, hematologic, and other methods. Studies of globin chain synthesis in vitro have contributed greatly to clarification of the basic underlying mechanism (1, 2, 24). This phenomenon of unequal rates of synthesis has two immediate consequences. First, there is a reduction or absence of synthesis of normal adult HbA ($\alpha_2\beta_2$). The production of HbF ($\alpha_2\gamma_2$) and Hb A_2 ($\alpha_2\delta_2$) continues but is inadequate to maintain a normal level of total red cell Hb. Second, there is an imbalance between α- and non-α-chain (β-, γ-, and δ-chains) production, with a net excess of α-chain synthesis, the α-chains being released uncoupled in the red cell. The α-chains are very instable and aggregate rapidly to form rigid and insoluble inclusions within the red cell [8]. This in turn causes damage to the red cell membrane, inhibition of erythroid maturation, premature cell destruction, and ineffective erythropoiesis [19, 20, 26].

The damage to red cell membrane involves increased permeability to potassium, with net loss of this intracellular cation; reduced ability to regenerate ATP; and a decrease in membrane plasticity [19, 20]. Membrane damage can also be caused by lipid peroxidation after the action of free radicals, which are generated in these defective cells [22]. The abnormal membrane function is more pronounced in the cells with a greater imbalance in globin synthesis; cells with relatively more γ-chain synthesis (i.e., HbF) have less membrane damage and longer survival [18].

In addition to the damage caused in the red cell membrane, α-chains seem to interfere with erythroid maturation. A great accumulation of early polychromatophilic erythroblasts with arrest in the G_1 phase of the cell cycle has been found in the bone marrow of β-thalassemic patients [26]. Autoradiographic studies have also shown that there is a defect in protein synthesis in the late erythroblasts [5].

These phenomena undoubtedly lead to ineffective erythropoiesis, with premature intramedullary death of these defective erythroblasts [5]. This ineffective erythropoiesis is the major factor responsible for the anemia of β-thalassemia.

A substantial proportion of thalassemic cells released from the bone marrow have a shortened survival, which has been attributed to the action of the excess α-chains in their cytoplasm. The mechanism by which excess α- chains result in shortened red cell survival is probably related to the transformation of these chains to irreversible inclusion bodies [7, 21]. The red cells are greatly distorted by these inclusion bodies and are trapped prematurely in the spleen, where many of them incur irreparable injury [19]. In other red cells, inclusion bodies may be removed by the sinusoids of the spleen, and the damaged red cells return to the circulation [13]. There is, however, a marked heterogeneity in the survival of red cells. Cells containing mainly HbA, free α-chains, and little HbF are short lived, whereas those having predominantly HbF survive longer [10, 19].

The ineffective erythropoiesis and the shortened red cell survival contribute to the development of the severe anemia of the disease. In accordance with the high oxygen affinity of the red cells due to the large amounts of HbF that they contain, this anemia produces severe tissue hypoxia, which constitutes a strong stimulus to erythropoietin production [12]. A massive increase in erythropoiesis results, with expansion of the erythroid bone marrow which spreads down the long bones and between the diploë. Occasionally, erythroid masses are found in areas not usually producting red cells, such as the maxilla, the orbit, and the frontal bone [29], or in extraosseous locations. However, in this greatly expanded erythroid bone marrow, most of the erythropoiesis is ineffective and cannot compensate for the anemia.

Marked erythroid hyperplasia also leads to a hypermetabolic state and increased need for folic acid [14]. Furthermore, the massively expanded erythron and ineffective erythropoiesis are probably responsible for the increased iron absorption. This, together with the blood transfusions given to these patients throughout their lives, results in iron overload. The iron has a special predilection for the endocrine glands, the liver, and the myocardium. How the iron damages these organs and causes fibrosis is not quite clear.

It can be concluded that the most devastating effect in β-thalassemia is the imbalance between α- and non-α-chain (especially β-chain) synthesis (β/α synthetic ratio). A "compensatory" synthesis of γ-chains occur which combine with free α-chains to form HbF ($\alpha_2\gamma_2$). Individuals with a high γ/α ratio have few α-chain inclusions and do better than individuals with a low γ/α ratio. Furthermore, the degree of anemia in β-thalassemia is dependent on the balance between excessive destruction of erythrocytes in the bone marrow or the spleen and the compensatory erythropoiesis.

The pathophysiology of β-thalassemia is summarized in Fig. 1. The heterozygous forms of β-thalassemia have a mild disorder with no or only mild anemia. This anemia has been attributed to ineffective erythropoiesis secondary to imbalance between α- and β-chain synthesis, which causes a small precipitation of α-chains [25].

α-Thalassemia

The pathophysiology of α-thalassemia is different from that of β-thalassemia. In α-thalassemia, the defect lies in the α-chain synthesis. This results in an excess of γ-chain production during the intrauterine and neonatal period, and of β-chains thereafter. However, unlike the α-chains, the β- and γ-chains do not precipitate significantly but form tetramers of β_4 (HbH) and γ_4 (HbBart's). These Hbs have a high oxygen affinity and lack the normal heme-to-heme

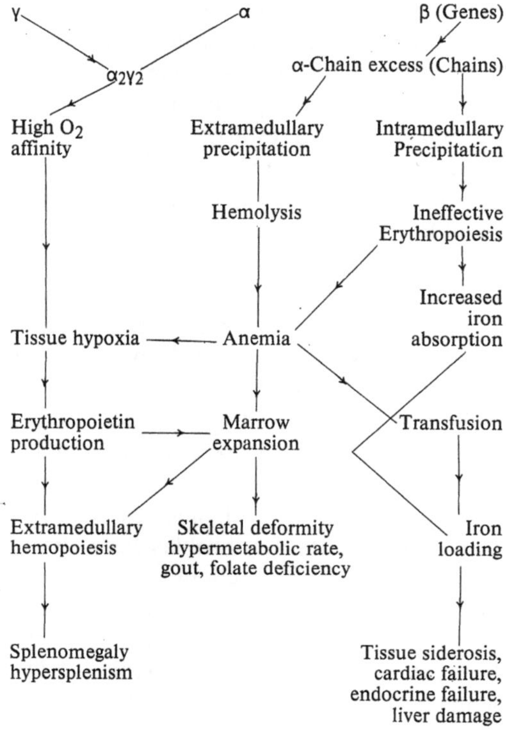

Fig. 1. The pathophysiology of β-thalassemia (from Williams WJ, Beutler E, Erslev AJ, Lichtman MA (1983) Hematology. McGraw-Hill, New York, p. 504)

interactions, which renders them physiologically useless.

α-Thalassemia occurs in four degrees of severity, depending on the number of deleted α-chains. Normal individuals inherit two α-chains from each parent. These four genes are found on the chromosome 16 pair. When all the α-globin genes are deleted no α-chains, and hence HbF ($\alpha_2\gamma_2$) can be made. Red cells are filled instead with HbBart's (γ_4), and death from tissue hypoxia is the inevitable outcome (hydrops fetalis). Dysfunction of three of the α-chains produces HbH disease, in which the β_4 tetramers (HbH) are unstable and are precipitated to form inclusion bodies of HbH [11]. These cells are prematurely destroyed by the spleen and the other organs of the monocyte-macrophage system, producing a mild anemia of hemolytic character. Varieties in which one or two α-genes are deleted are mild or asymptomatic.

Clinical and Laboratory Findings

β-Thalassemia

Initially before the genetic character of this disease was elucidated, the thalassemias were described according to their clinical severity, as already stated. Patients with major clinical manifestations and severe anemia were known as suffering from thalassemia major. Those patients with milder manifestations and anemia not necessitating regular transfusions were said to have thalassemia intermedia, whereas patients with little or no anemia but with characteristic abnormal erythrocytes were described as having thalassemia minor or minima [25, 27, 29].

Thalassemias are now described according to the globin chain (or chains) synthesized at a reduced rate and the homozygous or heterozygous condition of each case. We now know that thalassemia major comprises the severe homozygous condition, while thalassemia minor or minima comprises the heterozygous states. Thalassemia intermedia seems to result from the homozygous state of a mild form of β-thalassemia (e.g., β^{++}-thalassemia), from double heterozygosity of two different genes of β-thalassemia (e.g. $\beta^0/\delta\beta$-thalassemia), or from combination of β- with α-thalassemia gene [23].

Homozygous β-Thalassemia

In the majority of cases, the classical clinical syndrome of thalassemia major is produced by at least four genotypes: β^0/β^0, β^+/β^+, β^0/β^+, and $\delta\beta/\beta^0$. However, the clinical manifestations of all these variants are rather similar.

Classical β-thalassemia usually starts with severe anemia within the 1st year of life. Later, inadequately transfused children or children not treated at all develop the typical features of Cooley's anemia. Affected children fail to thrive and have all the signs and symptoms of severe anemia. Hepatosplenomegaly develops progressively, and mild jaundice may be present. Many features of a hypermetabolic state may develop, with anorexia, fever, and reduction of body weight; growth and maturation are retarded.

Characteristic bone changes occur, which are the result of expansion of the bone marrow cavities by the hyperactive erythroid mass. The most striking changes are seen in the skull and facial bones. The whole face gradually assumes a mongoloid appearance. A variety of other bone abnormalities develop, which are described elsewhere.

The above symptoms and signs are interspersed with frequent complications. These include recurrent infections, which are a common cause of death; spontaneous fractures due to expansion of the marrow cavities and thinning of the cortices; folic acid deficiency; hypersplenism due to gross splenomegaly; gallstones due to hyperbilirubinemia; and development of tumor masses resulting from the extramedullary hemopoietic tissue. There may be a bleeding tendency, which is associated with impaired hepatic synthesis of clotting factors.

The clinical course of the disease depends almost entirely on whether or not a regular transfusion regimen is started early in childhood. It should be remembered that the classical description of the disease by Cooley and others concerned children who were transfused inadequately or not at all. It is now well known that if transfusions are given soon enough, the affected children do not develop many of the "typical" features of the disease, grow normally, and present only a few of the complications of thalassemia. Clinical problems usually occur after the 1st decade and are the result of iron accumulation from the repeated blood transfusions, and perhaps increased iron absorption due to residual ineffective erythropoiesis.

Well-transfused children start to develop symptoms of iron overload as they enter puberty. Untreated children develop a similar clinical picture if they survive. The first indication of iron overload is the delay of pubescence and of secondary sex characteristics. Over the succeeding years, many other endocrine abnormalities develop, such as diabetes mellitus, adrenal insufficiency, hypoparathyroidism, hypothyroidism, and hypogonadism [3, 4, 9, 17]. Progressive liver damage is due to iron deposits, which involve the Kupffer cells, hepatocytes, and biliary epithelium, as in idiopathic hemochromatosis [29]. Cardiac complications arise early in the 2nd decade as a result of cardiac siderosis. Congestive heart failure and arrhythmias are the main clinical forms of cardiac involvement [6, 16].

Hematologic Features

There is always a severe degree of anemia. Prior to transfusions, Hb levels may be in the range of 0.02–0.06 g/ml. This anemia is typically hypochromic and microcytic. The red cells show marked anisopoikilocytosis, hypochromia, target cells, basophilic stippling, deformed microcytes, schistocytes, and occasional macrocytes. Erythroblasts are almost always present. The reticulocyte count is elevated (5%–15%), although less so than would be expected from the degree of anemia because of ineffective erythropoiesis. The white blood cells and platelets are normal or slightly elevated unless there is secondary hypersplenism.

The bone marrow is markedly hypercellular, with profound erythroid hyperplasia. The red cell precursors show defective Hb synthesis, as well as cytoplasmic inclusions of precipitated α-chains [7].

Iron kinetic studies indicate the presence of ineffective erythropoiesis and shortened red cell survival. It has been demonstrated that there are at least two populations of red cells - one which is rapidly destroyed and another with longer survival [15]. The short-lived population consists of red cells containing predominantly HbA, and the longer-surviving population contains relatively more HbF.

The osmotic fragility of the erythrocytes is markedly decreased. Some cells resist hemolysis in 0.1% saline solution.

The red cells of homozygous β-thalassemia have an increased level of HbF, ranging from 10% to more than 90%. In some cases, there is a complete absence of HbA, and the corresponding cells have only HbF and HbA_2. HbA_2 levels may be low, normal, or high according to the genetic form of thalassemia. In vitro Hb synthesis studies show imbalanced globin chain synthesis, with a marked excess of α- over β- and γ-chain synthesis.

β-Thalassemia Minor

This entity, which is also referred to as thalassemia trait, is rarely associated with significant clinical manifestations, except in periods of stress, such as pregnancy or severe infection, where a moderate degree of anemia may appear. The mean Hb level is about 15% lower than in normal persons of the same age and sex. Red cell morphology discloses some microcytosis, hypochromia, and poikilocytosis, with some target forms and basophilic stippling.

In most affected individuals, HbA_2 level increases to 3.5%–7%, while the level of HbF is slightly elevated in about half the patients. Hb electrophoresis, together with the osmotic fragility test, is useful in screening for heterozygous carriers in population surveys.

α-Thalassemia

As already stated, this kind of thalassemia comprises four clinical forms, distinguished according to the number of genes deleted. The most severe form of α-thalassemia is hydrops fetalis, which is due to deletion of all α-globin genes. This condition is incompatible with life, and affected infants either are delivered stillborn or die within the first few hours.

The HbH disease (three α-globin chains deleted) is a mild, well-compensated hemolytic anemia, with microcyte red cells which contain numerous inclusion bodies of HbH. HbA constitutes the major component on electrophoresis, while the level of HbH varies from 5% to 30%.

α-Thalassemia minor (two α-globin chains deleted) is a benign disorder characterized by morphologic alterations of the red cells and by the presence of HbBart's at birth, but with no significant hemolysis.

Finally, in the silent carrier state (one α-globin chain deleted), there are no clinical or hematologic abnormalities except for the demonstration of 1%–2% HbBart's in the affected neonates.

Summary

The pathophysiology and clinical and laboratory findings of the principal forms of thalassemia have been reviewed. The fundamental defect in β-thalassemia is reduction or absence of β-chain production, which results in an imbalance between α- and non-α-chain synthesis. α-chain precipitates in the red cell precursors create premature red cell destruction and ineffective erythropoiesis. The severe anemia which results causes a compensatory expansion of the erythroid mass, with skeletal deformities and a variety of metabolic abnormalities.

References

1. Bank A, Marks PA (1966) Excess α-chain synthesis relative to β-chain synthesis in thalassemia major and minor. Nature 212: 1198.
2. Bargellesis A, Pontremoli S, Menic C, Conconi F (1968) Excess of alpha globin synthesis in homozygous beta-thalassemia and its removal from the red cell cytoplasm. Eur J Biochem 3: 364
3. Costin G, Cocut MD, Human CB, Ortega JA (1977) Endocrine abnormalities in thalassemia major. Am J Dis Child 133: 497
4. Donabedia RK, Felig P, Genel M (1974) Endocrine evaluation in thalassemia major. Ann NY Acad Sci 232: 226
5. Dormer P, Betke K (1978) Erythroblasts kinetics in homozygous and heterozygous beta-thalassemia. Br J Haemat 38: 5
6. Engle MA (1964) Cardiac involvement in Cooley's anemia. Ann NY Acad Sci 119: 694
7. Fessas P (1963) Inclusions of hemoglobin in erythroblasts and erythrocytes of thalassemia. Blood 21: 21
8. Fessas P, Loukopoulos D (1974) The β-thalassemia. Clin Haematol 3: 411
9. Flynn DM, Fairney A, Jackson D, Cayton BA (1976) Hormonal changes in thalassemia major. Arch Dis Child 51: 828
10. Gabuzda TG, Nathan DG, Gardner FH (1963) The turnover of hemoglobins A, F and A_2 in the peripheral blood of three patients with thalassemia. J Clin Invest 42: 1678

11. Gabuzda TG (1966) Hemoglobin H and the red cell. Blood 27: 567
12. Hammond GD, Ishikawa A, Keighly G (1962) Relationship between erythropoietin and severe anemia in hypoplastic and hemolytic states. In: Jacobson LO, Doyle M (eds) Erythropoiesis. Grune and Stratton, New York
13. Jacob HS (1970) Mechanism of Heinz body formation and attachment to red cell membrane. Semin Hematol 7: 341
14. Jandl JH, Greenberg MS (1959) Bone marrow failure due to relative nutritional deficiency in Cooley's hemolytic anemia. New Engl J Med 266: 461
15. Kaplan E, Zuelzer WW (1950) Erythrocyte survival studies in childhood. II. Studies in Mediterranean anaemia. J Lab Clin Med 36: 517
16. Kremastinos DT, Toutouzas PK, Vyssoulis GP, Venetis CA, Avgoustakis DG (1984) Iron overload and left ventricular performance in β-thalassemia. Acta Cardiol (Brux) 39: 29
17. Livadas DP, Sofroniadou K, Souvatzoglou A, Boukis MA, Siafaka L, Koutras DA (1984) Functional insufficiency of thyroid and pituitary gland in beta-homozygous thalassemia with hemosiderosis. Acta Endorinol (Suppl) (Copenh) 265: 43
18. Loukopoulos D, Fessas P (1965) The distribution of hemoglobin types in thalassemic erythrocytes. J Clin Invest 44: 231
19. Nathan DG, Gunn RB (1966) Thalassemia: the consequence of unbalanced hemoglobin synthesis. Am J Med 41: 815
20. Nathan DG, Stossel TB, Gunn RB, Zarkowsky HS, Laforet MT (1969) Influence of hemoglobin precipitation on erythrocyte metabolism in alpha and beta thalassemia. J Clin Invest 48: 33
21. Rachmilewitz EA and Thorell B (1972) Hemochromes in single inclusion bodies in red cells of beta thalassemia. Blood 39: 794
22. Rachmilewitz EA (1976) The role of intracellular hemoglobin precipitation, low MCHC and iron overload on red blood cell membrane peroxidation in thalassemia. Birth defects 12: 123
23. Wainscoat JS, Kanavakis E, Wood WG, Letsky DJ, Huehns ER, Marsh GW, Higgs DR, Clegg JB, Weatherall DJ (1983) Thalassemia intermedia in Cyprus. The interactions of α and β thalassemia. Br J Haematol 53: 411
24. Weatherall DJ, Clegg JB, Naughton MA (1966) Globin synthesis in thalassemia. Nature 212: 1198
25. Weatherall DJ, Clegg JB (1981) The thalassemia syndromes. Blackwell Scientific, Oxford
26. Wickramasinghe SN, Letsky E, Moffatt (1973) Effect of α chain precipitates on bone marrow function in homozygous β thalassemia. Br J Haematol 25: 123
27. Williams WJ, Beutler E, Erslev AJ, Lichtman MA (1983) Hematology. McGraw-Hill, New York
28. Wintrobe MM (1981) Clinical hematology. Lea and Febiger, Philadelphia
29. Zaino EE (1980) Pathophysiology of thalassemia. Ann NY Acad Sci 344: 284

Part II
Imaging

4 Radiological Bone Changes in Thalassemia Major

Th. Cambouris

Introduction

The formation of blood cells in the fetus begins in the liver, spleen, thymus, and lymphatic tissue and finally extends into the bone marrow. In the infant and child, nearly all marrow spaces are engaged in active hematopoiesis. After completion of growth, blood cell production is limited to the proximal ends of the long bones, the vertebrae, and certain flat bones, all of which contain red marrow. The other marrow spaces contain largely yellow fatty tissue; however, they retain the ability to form new blood cells in times of exeptional need [5, 6, 8].

In severe anemia, the nonhematopoietic structures, including the fatty marrow, liver, and spleen, may become the source of red cell formation. If anemia is severe, long standing, and persistent, then there is marrow hyperplasia, which may be evident in the radiographic examination. The osseous changes of congenital hemolytic anemias are due primarily to overactivity and overgrowth of the hematopoietic marrow [2, 7].

This chapter describes the classical radiographic findings, i.e., radiographic findings for patients not adequately transfused. The X-ray skeletal changes in currently treated patients with β-thalassemia are described by Scutellari et al. [33; this volume].

Conventional radiography is the imaging procedure of choice in the initial work-up of bone lesions in patients with thalassemia major. Xeroradiography, radionuclide bone scans, computed tomography, and (recently) nuclear magnetic resonance are also generally effective for study of the skeletal system. Each skeletal imaging procedure contributes information with different sensitivity and specificity. Initially, skeletal lesions in patients with thalassemia major are evaluated by conventional films, which contribute considerable information concerning the nature and extent of the disease because they have not only an intermediate sensitivity but also high specificity [19, 25].

Xeroradiography

Xeroradiography represents a variation of conventional radiography. It is sometimes employed to diagnose a lesion because it is slightly more sensitive and has better resolution (1500 lines per inch) than X-ray films [12] (Fig. 2). Another advantage of xeroradiography is the accentuation of all edges of normal structures and pathological lesions so that they are more clearly demonstrated [34]. A third important characteristic is the wide contrast scale, which enables it to register small differences in tissue density with a high degree of detail. Simultaneous visualization of skin, subcutaneous fat, muscle, and bone is easily obtained [35]. The radiation dose for xeroradiography is significantly higher than that for similar examinations using film-screen technique.

Computed Tomography

If a skeletal lesion is suspected but conventional studies are not satisfactory, computed tomography is often the second choice [25]. It is used in practice as a problem-solving examination. It is not useful in the initial detection of a bone lesion and should not replace conventional radiography [3] (Fig. 4). Computed tomography has many advantages

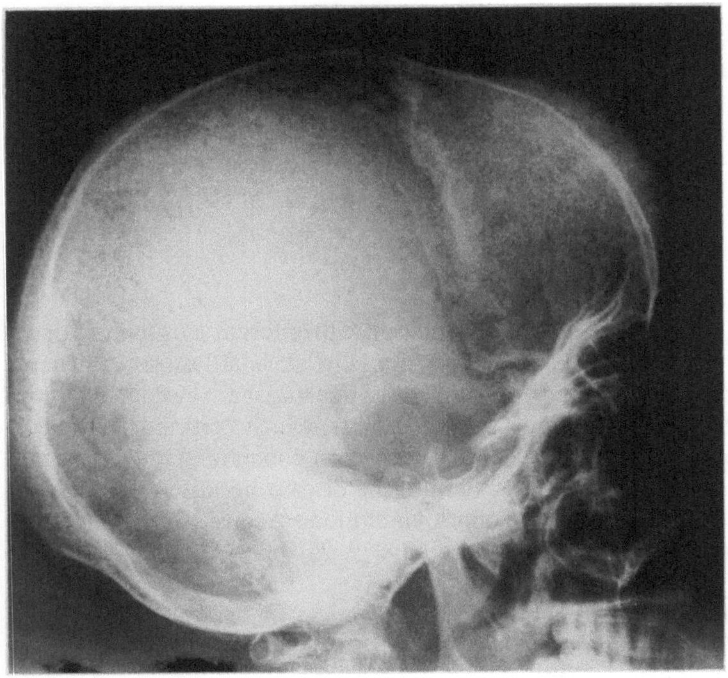

Fig. 1. Skull in thalassemia major. There is slight thickening of the diploë and thinning of the outer table. The bone structures are hazy and sandy due to generalized rarefaction

as an imaging technique, especially in thalassemic patients with marrow heterotopia (MH). It displays cross-sectional anatomy, and it can show the local extent of MH and its relationship to various structures [3].

Nuclear Magnetic Resonance

Nuclear magnetic resonance (NMR) is a new method of examination, which is promising in a number of musculoskeletal disorders. The excellent bony and soft-tissue contrast associated with the lack of ionizing radiation makes NMR an attractive method of examination in childhood. There are few reports which document the sensitivity of this method in identifying subtle changes in the composition of the medullary cavity in patients with various disorders [10].

Normally, the bone marrow gives a strong signal on NMR because of high fat content. In patients with β-thalassemia, there is a dramatic loss of normal high-intensity signal in the medullary cavity [26]. This probably reflects excessive iron deposition in the marrow or replacement of normal fatty marrow with fibrous tissue [26]. Other advantages of NMR are that it is not an invasive procedure, and that it can be repeated as often as needed.

In spite of these advantages, however, NMR cannot be established as a method of choice because it is an expensive and time-consuming procedure. In certain cases with MH, NMR may provide useful information (Fig. 24).

Radiological Changes

The radiological picture in severe cases of anemia is quite useful for diagnosis although when the changes are not so extreme, differentiation from the other types of hemolytic anemias is difficult. Radiographically, thalassemia major is identified by the diffuse bone changes which are caused by excessive proliferation of hemopoietic elements in the marrow space of the bones. The marrow cavity is notably widened and filled with red marrow tissue. However, the degree and severity of bone changes are often modified markedly as age increases. Not all bones of the skeleton

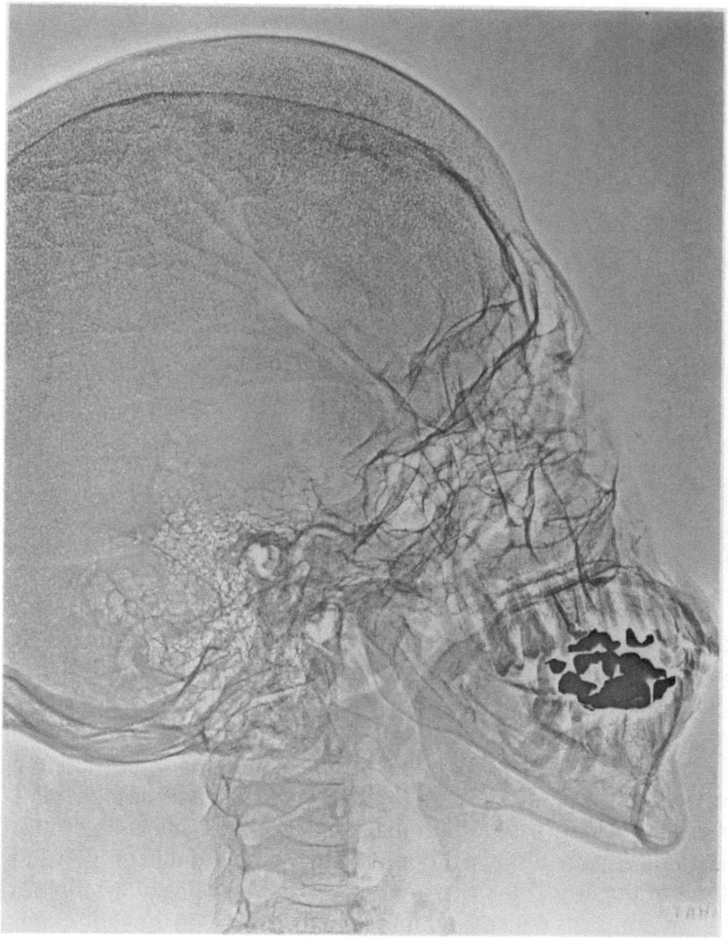

Fig. 2. Xeroradiogrpahy of skull in thalassemia major. There is generalized mottling throughout the calvarium due to osteoporosis. The diploic space is thick, mainly in the frontal bone. The grooves of the meningeal arteries are slightly enlarged

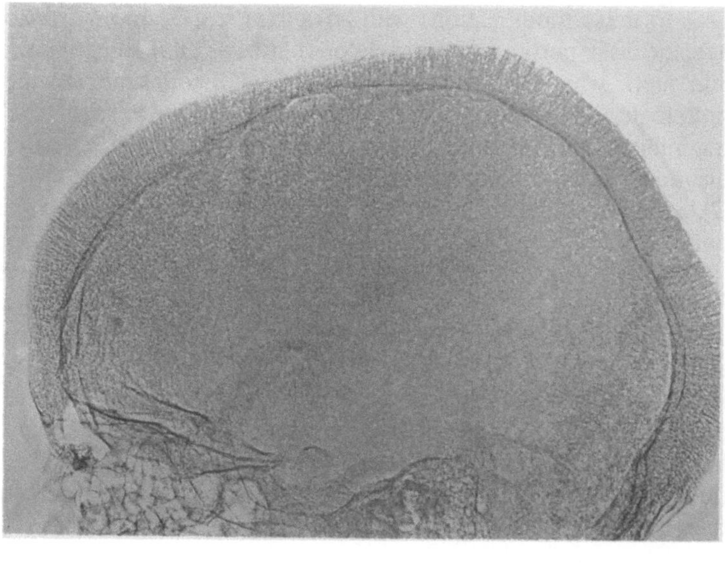

Fig. 3. Xeroradiography of skull in thalassemia major. There is generalized osteoporosis, associated with numerous striations perpendicular to the inner table, which is thin but preserved

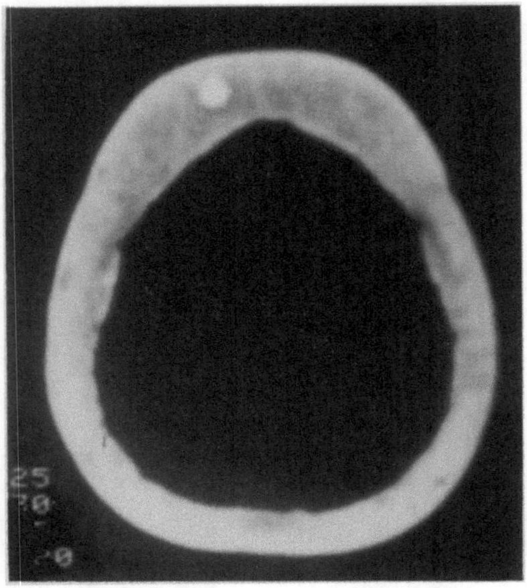

Fig. 4. Computerized tomogram of skull (window for bones) in a patient with thalassemia major. There is marked thickening of the diploic space, which is about four times the normal width. The outer and inner tables are sharply demarcated. Note the deep vascular notchings of the inner table

are afflicted to the same degree. The radiological findings for the skull do not always run parallel to the changes in the rest of the skeleton or to the degree of anemia [32]. As it has been mentioned, in the peripheral parts of the skeleton where the normally red marrow is replaced by fatty tissue, the initial radiographic changes may disappear completely by the time of puberty [28].

In contrast, the radiographic changes in the skull, spine, and pelvis persist throughout life or may even become more pronounced. Due to these modifications with advancing age, the distal portions of the skeleton (hands and feet), which are the optimal sites for radiological identification of the disease during infancy and childhood, become the least diagnostic after puberty according to Caffey [7], as the bone lesions regress during childhood.

Skull

The changes in the skull are quite distinctive and more common in Cooley's anemia than in the other congenital anemias. It must be pointed out that the skull changes represent a late skeletal manifestation of the disorder. In mild cases, X-rays may show only a slight thickening of the vault, with increased porosity. Radiographically, the bones may be somewhat hazy and sandy (Fig. 1). At a later stage, the bones assume a more spongy outline, due to mottling throughout their medullary portion (Fig. 2). As the disease progresses, there is a notable thinning of the inner table and disappearance of the outer table of the vault, with a concurrent thickening of the diploë (Fig. 3). The earliest changes in the skull occur most commonly in the frontal bone, but the parietal and temporal bones are also involved [7, 27]. Feingold and Case [17] have described several cases in which after thickening the diploë was as much as four times as wide as the normal bone (Fig. 4). Due to asymmetrical thickening of the diploic space, the calvarium may assume a camelback shape (Fig. 5). Very often, the hyperplastic marrow perforates or destroys the outer table, which becomes so thin as to be indistinguishable, while the inner table remains intact [7, 28] (Figs. 5, 6). At times, diploic new bone spicules are laid down perpendicularly to the inner table, producing the characteristic radial pattern, with a "hair-standing-on-end" appearance [7, 27, 36] (Fig. 7). The radiating spicules are easily recognized when tangential roetgenographic projections of the skull are studied [19] (Fig. 8); however, they

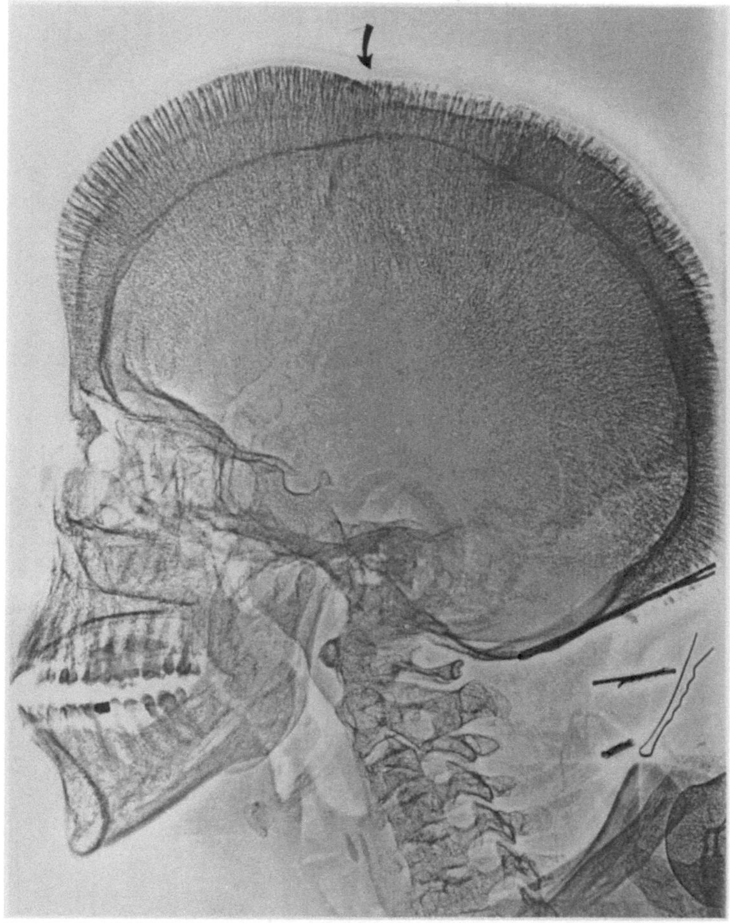

Fig. 5. Xeroradiography of skull in a patient with severe thalassemia major. There is marked widening of the diploic space, mainly in the frontal bone, which is asymmetric and uneven, giving a camelback appearance (*arrow*). New bone spicules are laid down perpendicular to the inner table, producing the characteristic hair-on-end appearance. Note the lack of changes in the occipital squamosa, inferior to the internal occipital protuberance

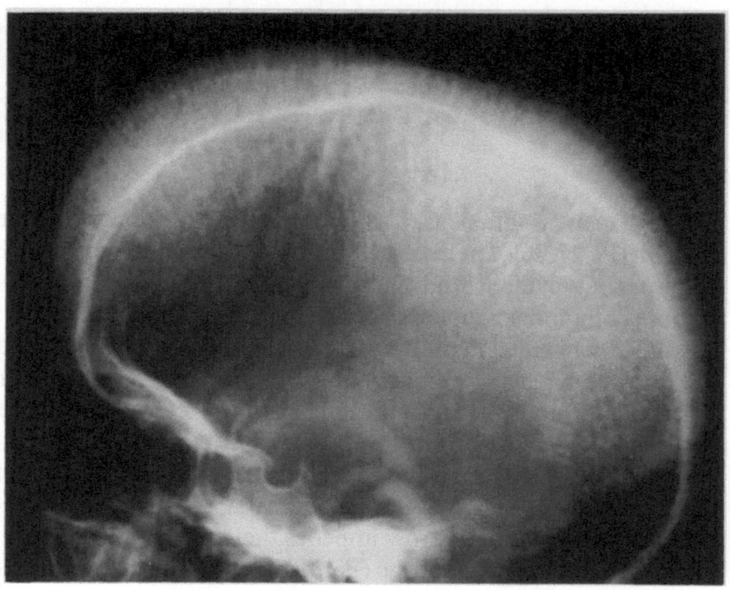

Fig. 6. Skull in thalassemia major. The diploic space is considerably widened in the frontal, parietal, and occipital bones. Hyperplastic marrow has perforated the outer table; the inner table remains intact. All bones show a granular osteoporosis

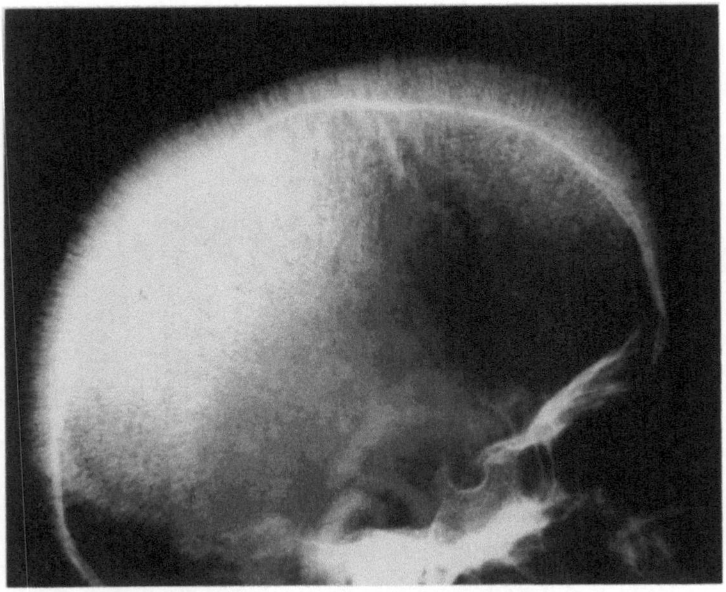

Fig. 7. Skull in thalassemia major. The entire vault except for the squamous occiput is seriously affected by the disease. There are multiple radiating spicules perpendicular to the inner table of the skull caused by hyperplastic marrow, giving a hair-on-end appearance. The inner table is well defined; the outer table lacks definition

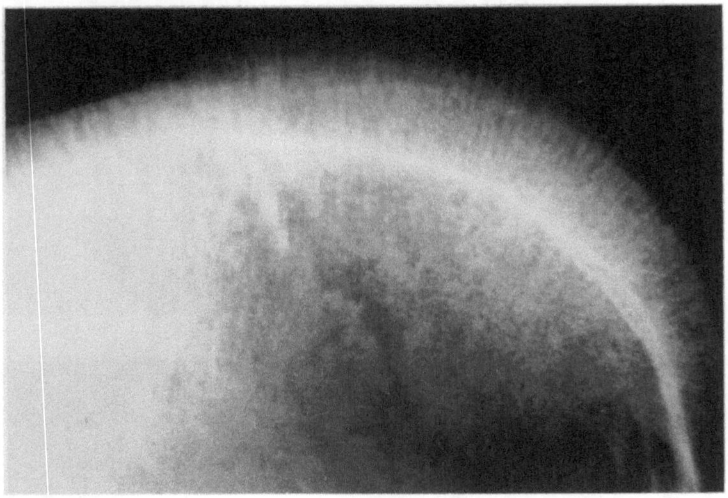

Fig. 8. Skull in a patient with severe thalassemia major: close-up of the frontal bone. Note the coarse radial spicules perpendicular to the inner table, which produce the characteristic hair-on-end appearance

are not seen as often as it is commonly thought [19, 27, 36]. The classical hair-on-end pattern is only evident in advanced stages and is more common in Cooley's anemia than in any other congenital hemolytic anemia. The middle meningeal grooves are often enlarged, tortuous, elongated, and sharply delineated [24] (Fig. 9).

Marrow hyperplasia is prominent also in the facial bones [1, 2, 5, 6]. In the paranasal bones, overgrowth of marrow impedes their pneumatization at an early age (Fig. 10 a–c). Although pneumatization of the cranial sinuses is retarded to a marked degree in all patients not all sinuses are afflicted to the same degree [17]. Lack of pneumatization in the maxillary and sphenoidal sinuses is most consistent and more marked than in the ethmoidal sinuses. According to Caffey [7], the noninvolvement of the ethmoidal sinuses is due to the fact that there is little marrow activity or even no marrow space in the ethmoidal bones (Fig. 11 a, b). Changes in the sinuses are not usually seen in other anemias.

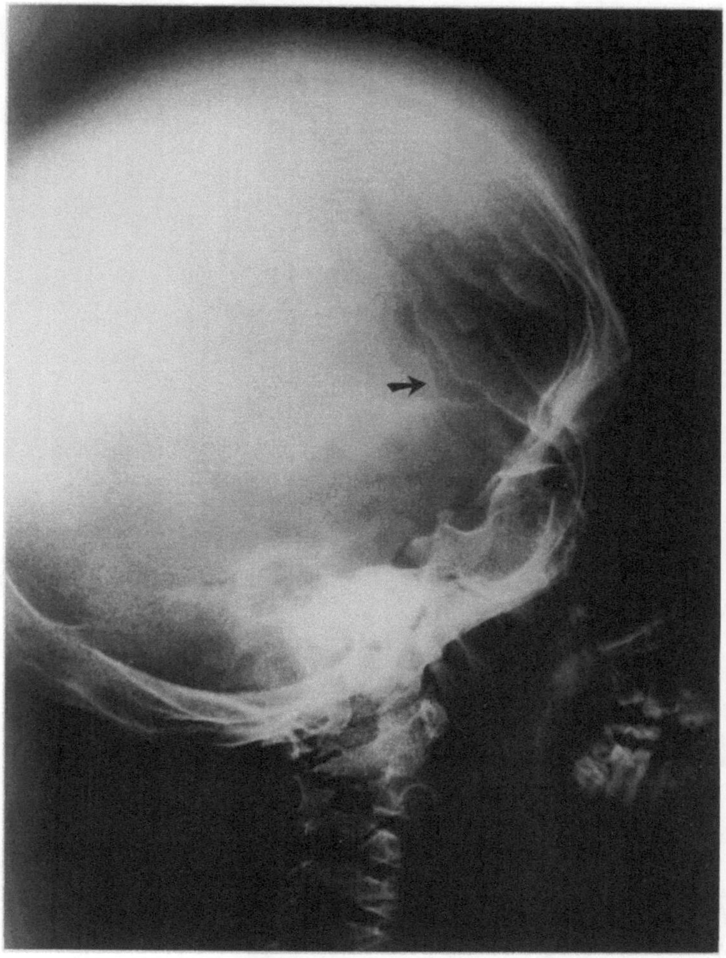

Fig. 9. Skull in thalassemia major. The middle meningeal groove is quite enlarged, tortuous, elongated, and sharply defined (*arrow*). There is also slight thickening of the diploic space. Pneumatization of the mastoids is suppressed

In the temporal bones, marrow activity varies considerably between individuals, so that pneumatization may be normal, slightly suppressed, or completely suppressed [7] (Fig. 10 a–c).

The degree of involvement of the frontal sinuses is somewhat difficult to estimate since pneumatization of this structure normally shows wide variations. In his classic description of Cooley's anemia, Caffey [7] pointed out: There is usually a conspicuous lack of bone thickening in the occipital squamosa below the internal occipital protuberance. This is a fortunate circumstance because marked thickening of the edges of the foramen magnum would lead inevitably to compression of the underlying channels of the cerebrospinal fluid flow and/or the central nervous system itself. This segment of the occipital squamosa is probably deficient in marrow.

The disproportionate marrow overgrowth of the upper maxilla leads to swelling of this bone, overbite of the mandible, and malocclusion of the jaw [20]. As a result of this deformity, the upper central incisors protrude ventrally, thus giving rise to the so-called rodent face [6, 7, 11]. This is a distinctive pathognomonic sign of Cooley's anemia, especially when it is associated with non pneumatization of the paranasal sinuses. Marked hypertrophy of the upper maxilla may also in some patients be the cause of displacement of the orbits laterally, producing

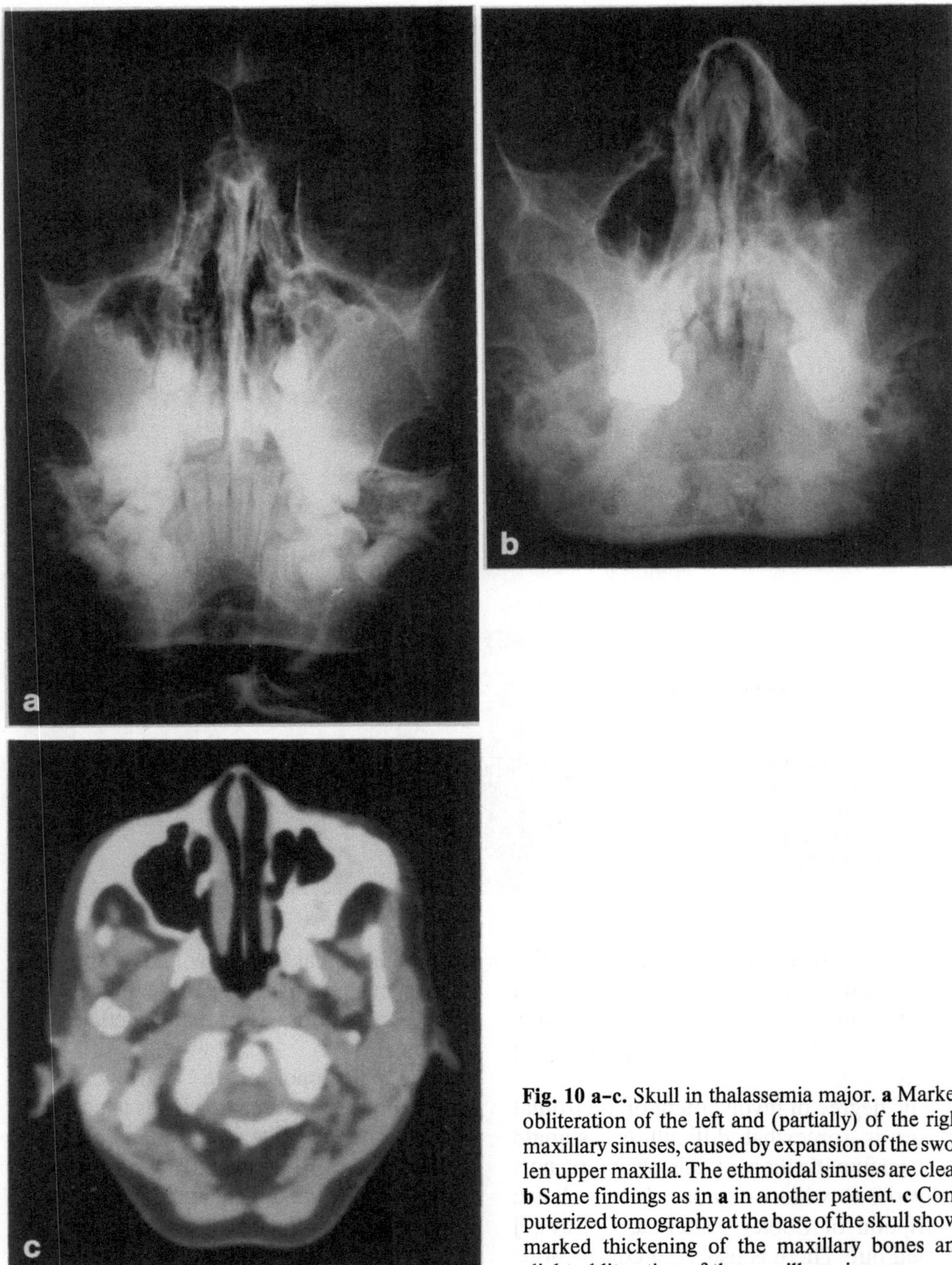

Fig. 10 a–c. Skull in thalassemia major. **a** Marked obliteration of the left and (partially) of the right maxillary sinuses, caused by expansion of the swollen upper maxilla. The ethmoidal sinuses are clear. **b** Same findings as in **a** in another patient. **c** Computerized tomography at the base of the skull shows marked thickening of the maxillary bones and slight obliteration of the maxillary sinuses

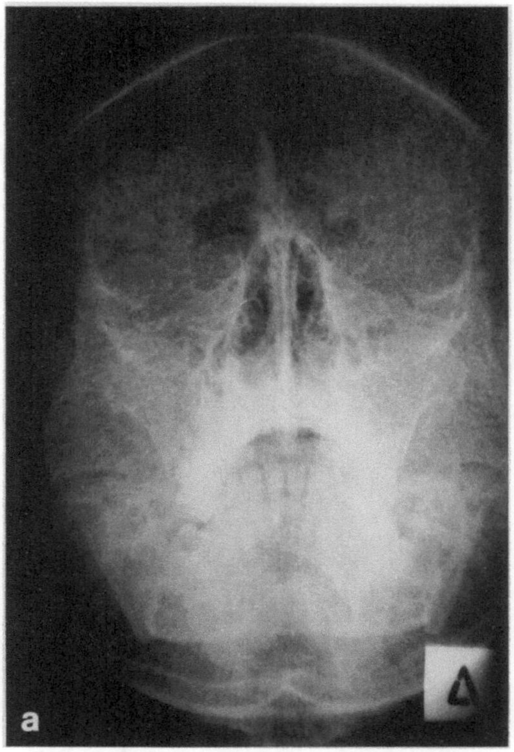

Fig. 11 a, b. Skull (facial bones) in thalassemia major. **a.** Lack of pneumatization of the maxillary sinuses and (partially) of the left frontal sinus. All facial bones are markedly thickened and show typical coarse trabeculation. The ethmoidal sinuses are characteristically free of involvement. **b.** Xeroradiograph showing generalized sandy osteoporosis and overgrowth of the maxillary bones, which impairs the paranasal sinuses. The ethmoidal sinuses are not involved

marked ocular hypertelorism due to increase of the interorbital distance [11].

Small Tubular Bones

The small tubular bones of the hands and feet are the optimal sites for an earlier radiological demonstration of Cooley's anemia in infants and children since red marrow is found in the entire skeleton in this age group. Marrow hyperplasia in the short tubular bones causes medullary widening and thinning of the cortex because of pressure atrophy (Fig. 12). Small, cystlike lucencies or cortical erosive defects may develop in the hands or feet (Fig. 13 a, b). The spongiosa is sparse, and in some instances it may almost disappear, giving the picture of osteoporosis [7, 27]. In most typical cases, however, there is a coarse trabeculation in the shafts of the short tubular bones (Fig. 14). This is due to absorbtion and/or destruction of the fine trabeculae because of marrow hyperplasia. Consequently, new bone is laid down on the remaining trabeculae, thus making them thicker. On the other hand, the concurrent thinning of the cortex makes the remaining, thickened trabeculae more conspicuous than normal [19, 27, 36]. Marrow hypertrophy also bulges out the normally concave contour of the shafts. The small tubular bones become wider than normal and lose their concavity, and the metacarpals, metatarsals, and phalanges assume a rectangular appearance (Fig. 15). Such changes may also be found in other diseases in which overstimulation of the bone marrow occurs early in life, when the bones are young and relatively elastic and expansible [2, 11, 27, 36].

Another finding which might be encountered in patients with thalassemia major is enlargement of the nutrient foramina in the hands. This may most probably be due to the increased need for blood supply of the hypertrophied bone morrow. The size of the foramina usually varies from 1 to 2 mm [18, 24]. Radiographically, the enlarged nutrient

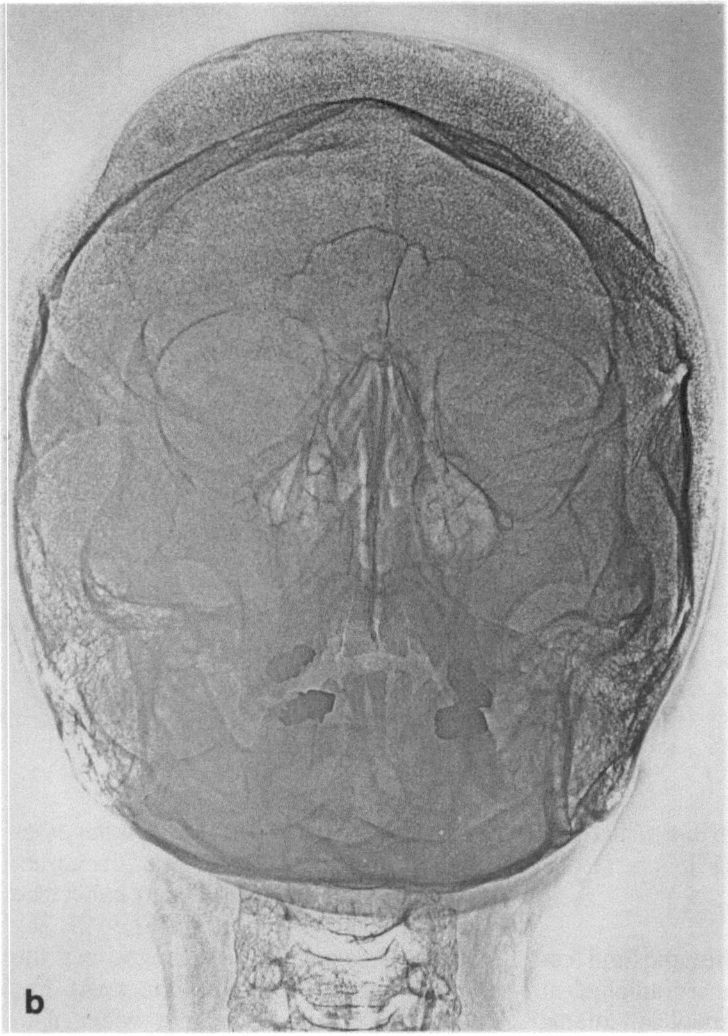

Fig. 11 b

foramina are shown as round or oval lucencies in the center of the metacarpals or phalanges, usually nearer to the distal ends (Fig. 16 a, b). This finding is not pathognomonic of β-thalassemia because it may also be encountered in patients with Gaucher's disease.

Long Bones

Transverse bands of increased density (growth lines) may be observed across the metaphyseal portions of the long bones in children with thalassemia major. They may persist in adult life, and they do not have any clinical significance (Fig. 17 a, b). The long bones may also lose their normal contour and appear "swollen" due to widening of the medullary canal as a result of marrow hypertrophy, which consequently causes pressure atrophy of the cortex [19, 36]. The coarse hypertrophied pattern may assume a characteristic generalized cystlike appearance, which becomes radiographically more conspicuous due to the coexistent cortical atrophy (Fig. 18 a, b).

Spine

The vertebral bodies in patients with thalassemia major are of an average size, but they

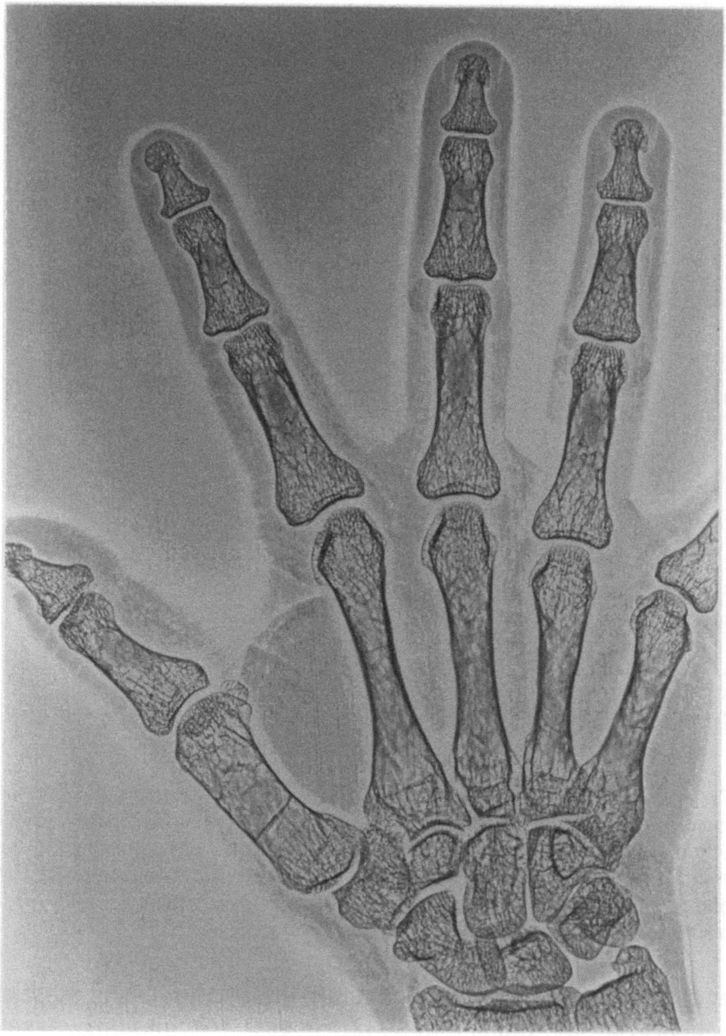

Fig. 12. Hand in thalassemia major. The trabecular pattern of the metacarpals and phalanges is prominent with thinning of the cortex because of pressure atrophy. The medullary cavities of the phalanges are slightly widened

present slight bulging of their contour (Fig. 19). There is a diffuse demineralization, with a coarsened reticulation of the vertebral bodies, which is also evident in the pedicles, the laminae, and the transverse and spinous processes [16] (Fig. 20). The surviving trabeculae of the vertebral bodies are arranged vertically (Fig. 21 a, b). The steplike defect which is characteristic of sickle cell anemia is practically never seen in thalassemia. In advanced cases of thalassemia, vertebral coolapse may occur. There is no deformity of the neural arches or intervertebral foramina. Over the years, the vertebral bodies grow normally in size and appearance [9, 16].

Ribs

Rib changes are often observed in patients with thalassemia. The findings vary according to the age when the transfusion regimen is started. Delayed or low transfusion regimen is associated with widening of the ribs, which is explained by the marked compensatory marrow hypertrophy and subsequent expansion and thinning of the cortex [22, 27]. It is believed that rib changes can be prevented it hypertransfusion regimes begin early in life. Frequent blood transfusions may partially alleviate the demands on the bone marrow; this explains the relative infrequency of rib changes and perhaps the lack of intrathoracic

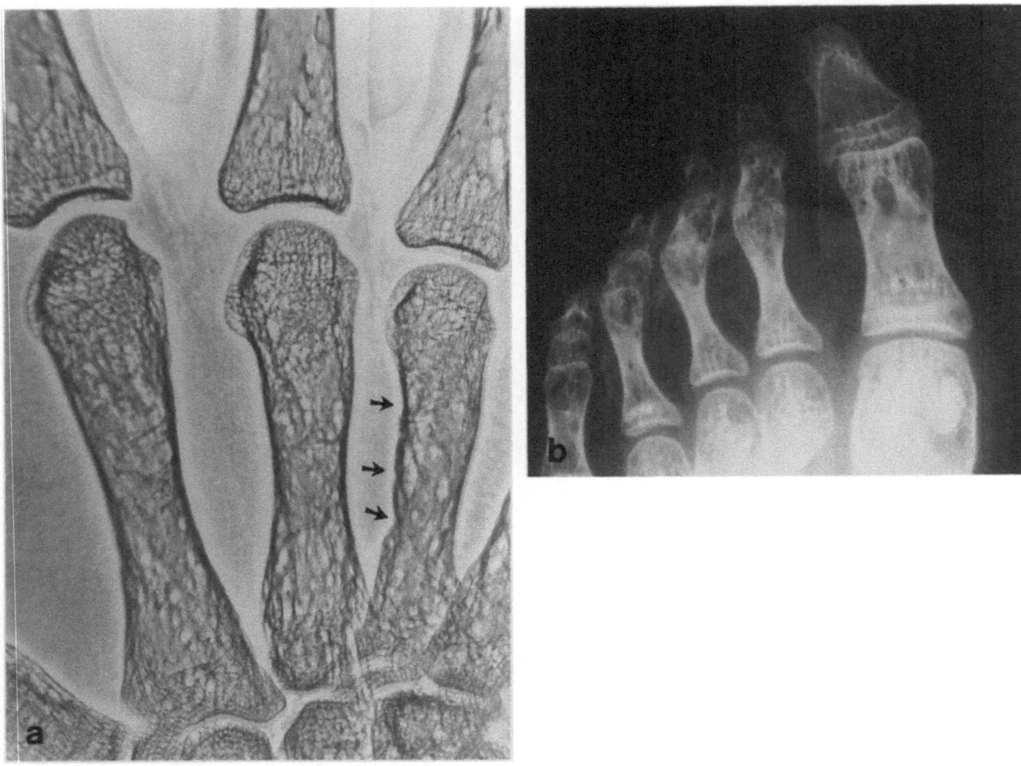

Fig. 13a, b. Hand and foot in severe thalassemia major. **a** Xeroradiograph of hand. Note the cortical thinning and erosion of the metacarpals (*arrows*), associated with a coarse trabecular pattern because of marrow hyperplasia. There is also some deviation from normal tubulation. The localized areas of lucencies are due to tumorous collection of hyperplastic marrow. **b** Coarse trabecular pattern of the distal phalanges of the foot. Note the cystlike lucencies in toes, caused by focal collection of hyperplastic marrow

extramedullary hemopoiesis among these patients [27, 30]. Lawson et al. [22] noticed regression of abnormal findings in two-thirds of their patients after the onset of a hypertransfusion regimen.

The most common finding is widening of the ribs associated with osteoporosis and a characteristic trabeculated pattern involving their entire length (Fig. 22). The cortex is usually thin and atrophic. In addition, small, localized, well-defined lucencies (1 or 2 mm in size) can be seen in the medulla [22, 27].

Expansion is more often seen in the posterior than in the anterior end of the rib (Fig. 23). Posterior rib expansion may lead to thoracic extramedullary hemopoiesis [14, 21, 30, 31] (Fig. 24 a, b). Marked medullary rib expansion has been described by some authors in other entities, e.g., in diffuse neuroblastoma, Niemann-Pick disease, and leukemia [27].

Notching is occasionally found along the inferior margin of the posterior portion of the ribs, and it may mimic the erosions produced by coarctation of the aorta or neurofibromas (Fig. 25). Notching can also be found in the upper margin of the posterior ends of the ribs [4, 15, 22]. According to Moseley [27], these irregular rib indentations are the effect of subperiosteal marrow proliferation rather than of vascular defects.

Another relatively common rib change is the presence of a line of increased density extending across the medullary space of the rib, parallel to its long axis. This is best seen in the anterior portions of the ribs [22, 27], and it

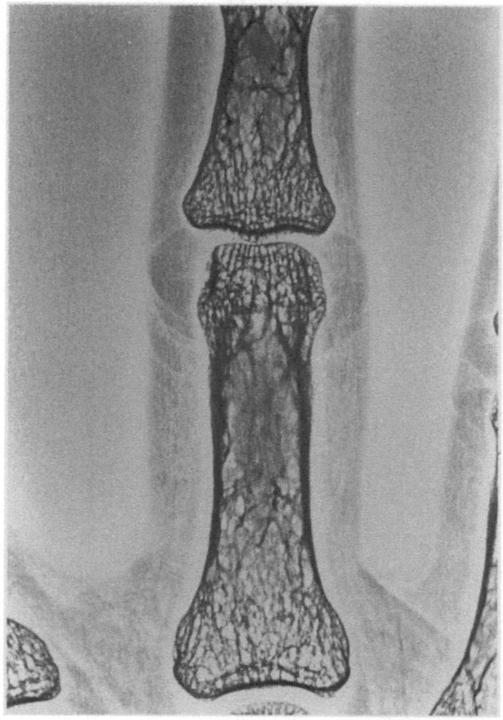

Fig. 14. Close-up of phalanx in a patient with thalassemia major, showing cortical atrophy, swollen external contour, rarefaction, and coarse trabeculation

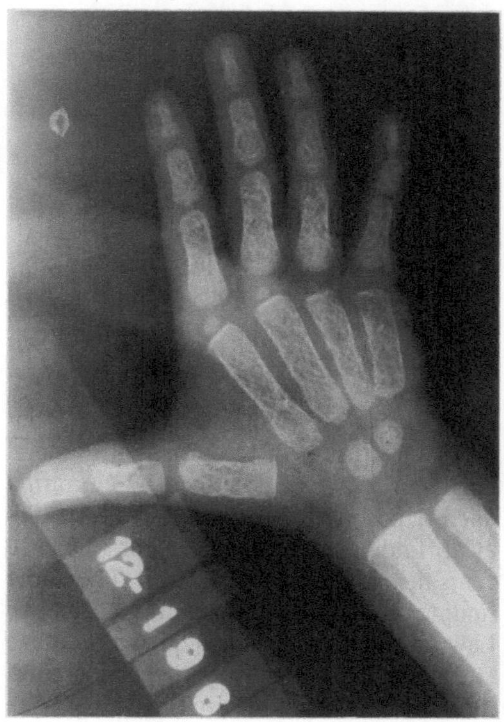

Fig. 15. Hand in severe thalassemia major. Coarse trabeculation is seen in the metacarpals and phalanges, which form a honeycomb pattern. The fingers appear to be swollen due to pressure of the expanding marrow space. The cortices are thinned. Note the absence of modeling in metacarpals and phalanges, which tend to assume a rectangular shape. The small localized lucencies represent collections of hyperplastic marrow

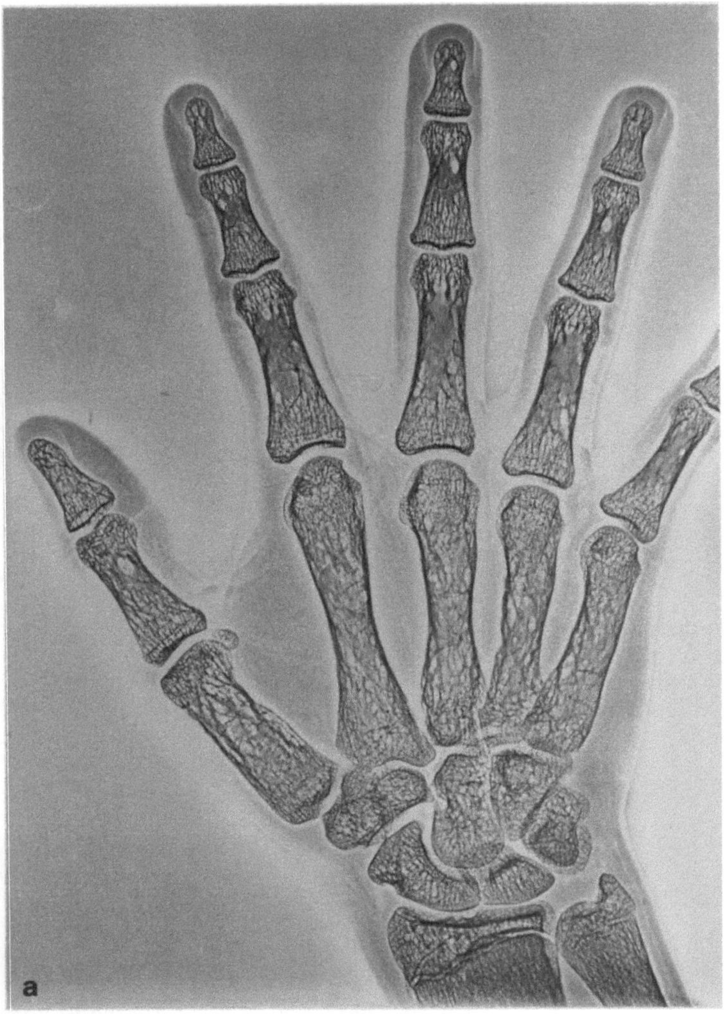

Fig. 16 a, b. Xeroradiograph of Hand in thalassemia major. **a** Coarse trabecular pattern of marrow associated with cortical thinning and cortical erosive defects in the first, fourth, and fifth metacarpal bones. The nutrient foramina in the middle phalanges are enlarged and well defined. **b** Close-up of hand in **a**. The enlarged nutrient foramina are demonstrated as round or oval punched-out lucencies in the middle and distal phalanges, the diameter of which varies from 1 to 3 mm

has been described as "rib within the rib." This sign has also been observed in cases of sickle cell anemia, but it is more common in thalassemia major [19, 22, 27].

Early Fusion of Epiphyses

Premature fusion of the proximal humeral epiphyses was first described by Currarino and Erlandson [13] as a characteristic radiological finding in patients older than 10 years,the incidence being 14%. The same finding was described and confirmed later by Lawson and his colleagues [23]. According to Currarino and Erlandson [13], the most common site of fusion is the proximal end of one or both humeri and the distal end of one or both femurs. The tibia can also be affected, but only very rarely. The fusion tends to involve only a segment of the epiphyseal plate rather than its entire width. In the humerus, premature fusion almost always involves the medial segment of the proximal epiphyseal plate [13].

In patients in whom the epiphyseal lines are still open, the segmental location of the fusion can be demonstrated radiographically. It appears as an area of bone sclerosis crossing and bridging the epiphyseal line at the site of the early fusion. As a result of this fusion, there is some degree of shortening of the

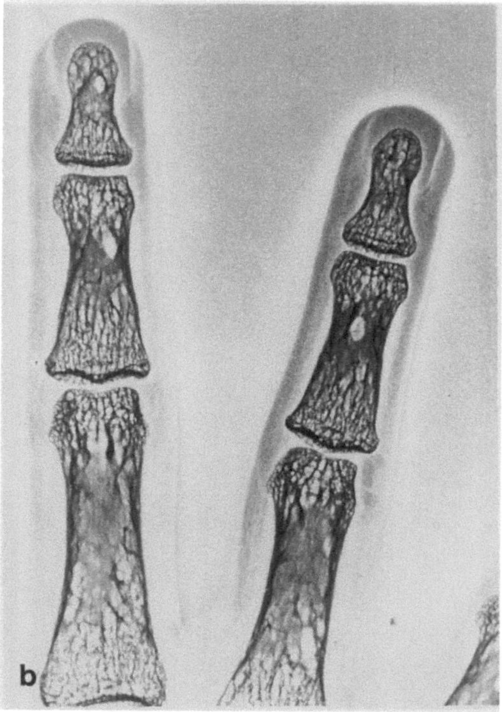

Fig. 16 b

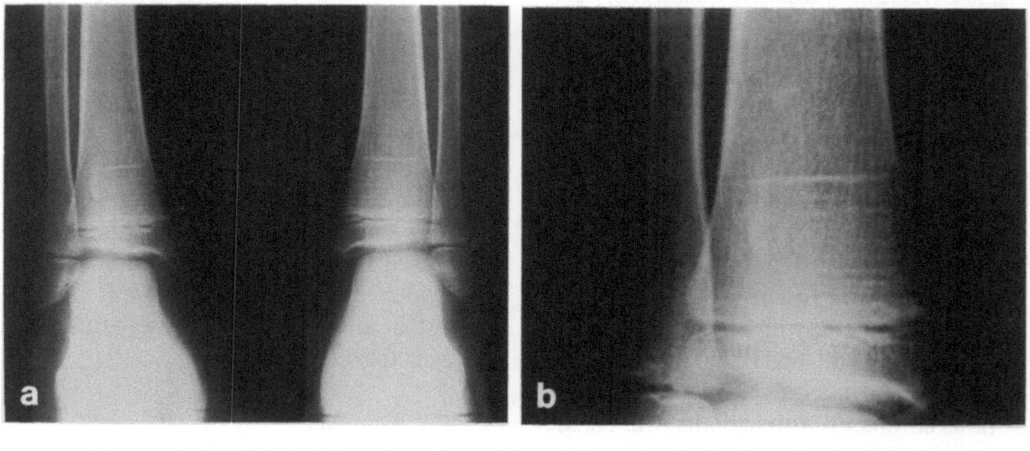

Fig. 17 a, b. Lower legs in thalassemia major. **a** Growth lines symmetrically distributed at the metaphyseal portions of both tibiae. **b** Close-up of tibia of the patient in **a**

affected bone and a bony deformity of the involved area [13, 23]. The shortening is more obvious in the humeri than in femurs. In older patients, in whom all the epiphyseal lines are obliterated, the appearance of the bony deformity or shortening suggests that the abnormal fusion was originally also segmental in location (Fig. 26 a, b).

In bones of which the segmental fusion is eccentrically situated, the deformity is characterized by a tilt of the epiphysis toward the site of fusion. In fact, in the humerus the

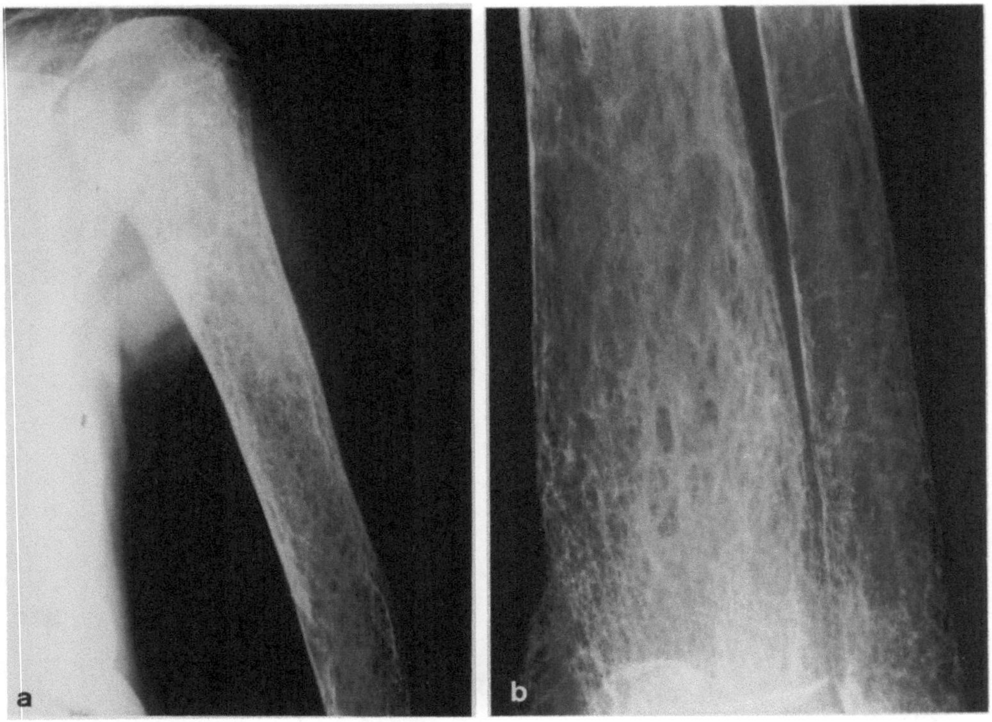

Fig. 18 a. Humerus in thalassemia major. The humerus has lost its normal contours and appears to be swollen due to marrow hypertrophy. The cortex is thin. The mottled osteoporosis and hypertrophied trabeculae result in a generalized cystlike appearance. **b.** Tibia and fibula in thalassemia major. There is marked thinning of the cortices of tibia and fibula, associated with accentuation of the bony trabecular pattern, also producing a cystlike appearance (like a sponge)

epiphysis is tilted medially, while in the femurs it is tilted posteriorly or anteriorly, according to the position of fusion (Fig. 27).

Currarino and Erlandson [13] noted that 26% of their patients with premature fusion of the epiphyses had thalassemia intermedia. These patients had only a few or no transfusions as compared with patients with talassemia major. The higher incidence of premature fusion of the epiphyses in patients with thalassemia inermedia was attributed by the same authors not to the severity of the disease - and in particular not to the number of previous blood transfusions - but to the fact that these patients live longer than those with thalassemia major.

Lawson et al. [23] reported that 7 of their 17 patients with premature fusion of the epiphyses had thalassemia intermedia; these patients had never been transfused. In contrast, 12 of their patients who were hypertransfused from an early age did not reveal any evidence of premature fusion. It must be noted that all but one of their patients were younger than 10 years old.

Aseptic Necrosis

Aseptic necrosis of the femoral head as a complication of homozygous β-thalassemia has been reported recently by Orzincolo et al. [29]. These authors described 4 cases of aseptic necrosis of the femoral head in a group of 280 thalassemic patients. They emphasized that the frequency of this complication was higher in homozygous β-thalassemic patients (1,4%) than in the normal population (0.1%).

The X-ray findings are those usually seen in Legg-Calvé-Parthes disease, i.e., subcorti-

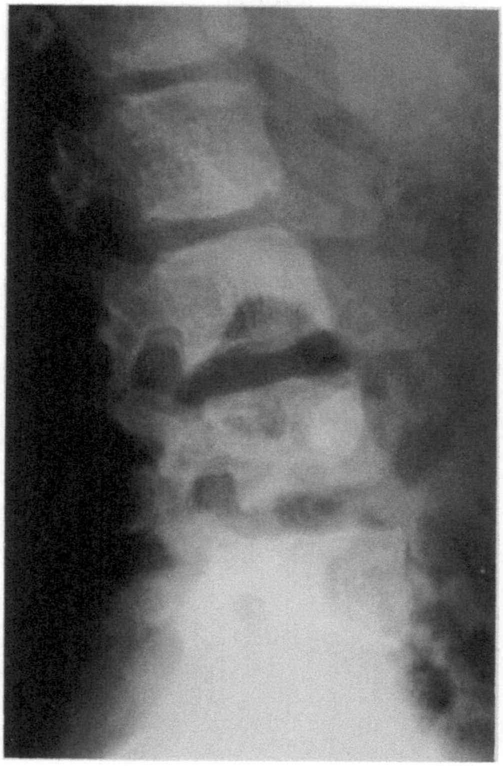

Fig. 19. Lumbar spine in thalassemia major. The size of the vertebral bodies is normal, but they demonstrate a slight bulging of the contour. There is also slight demineralization and coarsened trabeculation

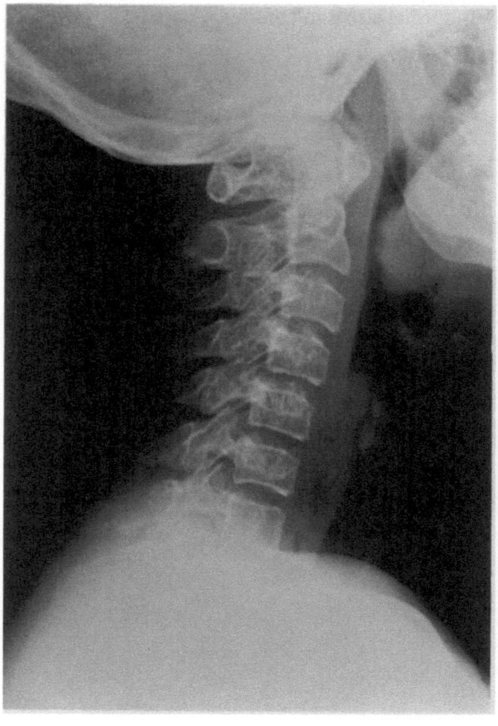

Fig. 20. Cervical spine in thalassemia major. The spine shows a diffuse, coarsened trabecular pattern. All parts of the vertebral bodies (spinous processes, laminae, etc.) become osteoporotic. Compression deformities may occur occasionally

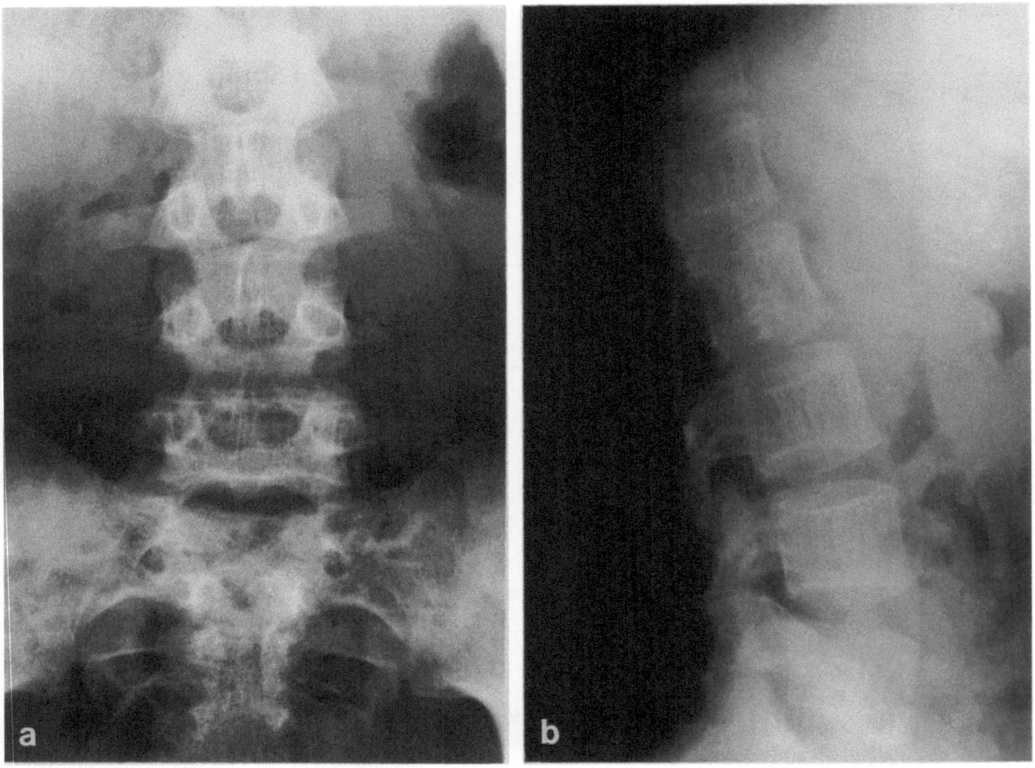

Fig. 21 a, b. Lumbar spine in thalassemia major, face (**a**) and profile (**b**). The vertebral bodies maintain their normal size and contour. There is, however, a coarse perpendicular pattern associated with osteoporosis. The biconcavity commonly seen in sickle cell syndromes is not present in thalassemia major

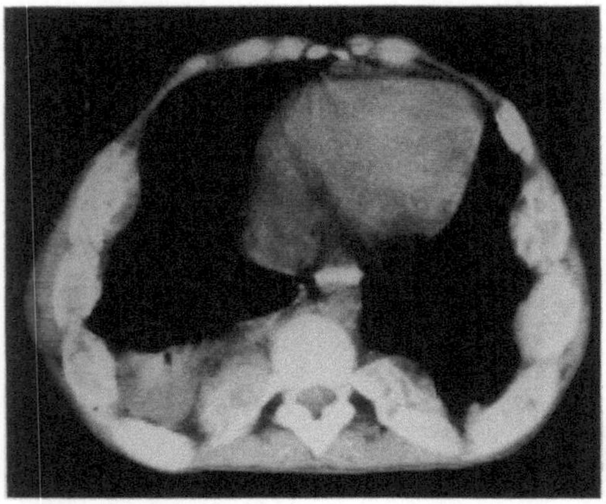

Fig. 22. Computerized tomogram of the thorax in thalassemia major (window for bones) at the level of the heart. It shows extramedullary hemopoiesis and marked thickening of the ribs

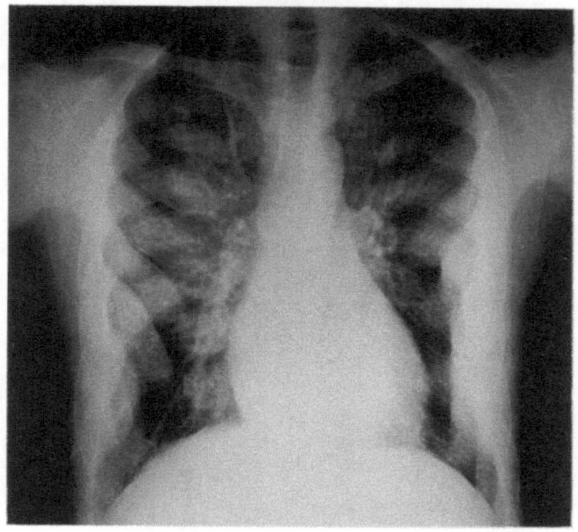

Fig. 23. Ribs in thalassemia major. All ribs are markedly swollen not only posteriorly but mainly anteriorly, forming masses which have been described as a "fingerlike" pattern. There is also diffuse osteoporosis and thinning of the cortices

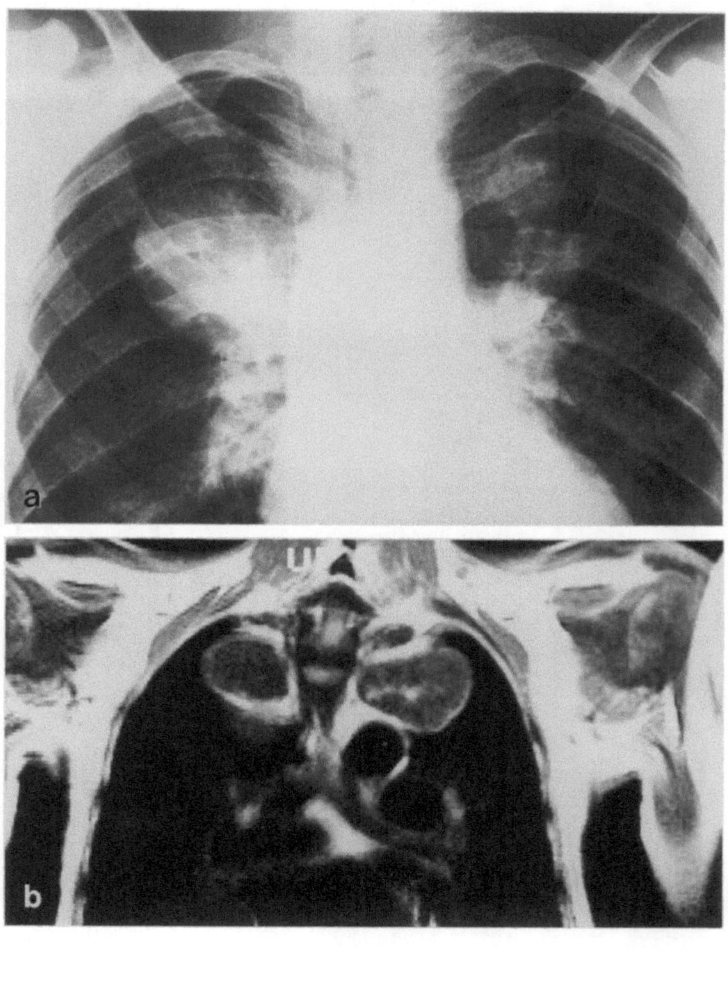

Fig. 24 a, b. Chest in thalassemia major. **a** Frontal view demonstrates lobulated posterior mediastinal masses of hemopoietic tissue in the middle thoracic region, especially on the right side. **b** Coronal section (NMR, T_1-weighted image). The extramedullary masses appear as ring lesions in the paravertebral space, with bright rim and low-intensity center. The left lesion shows linear increased intensity attributed to deposition of fat. In front of the lesion, the normal aortic knob is noted

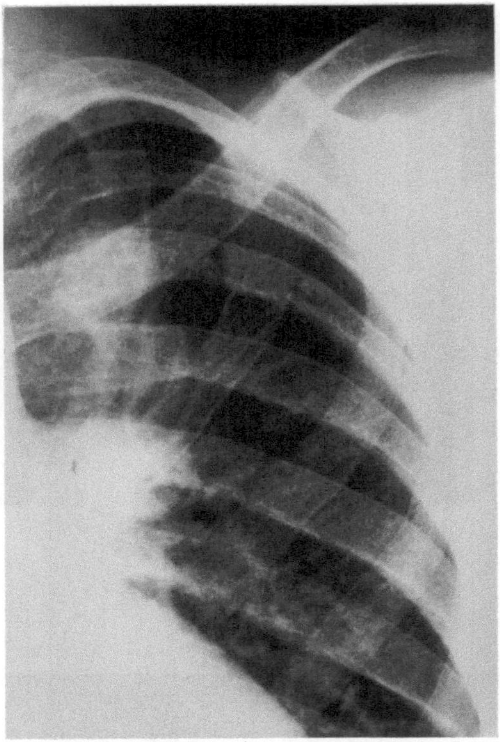
25

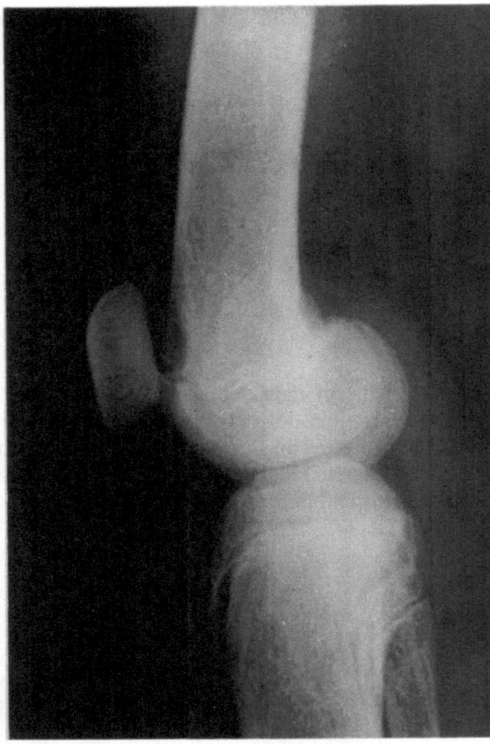
27

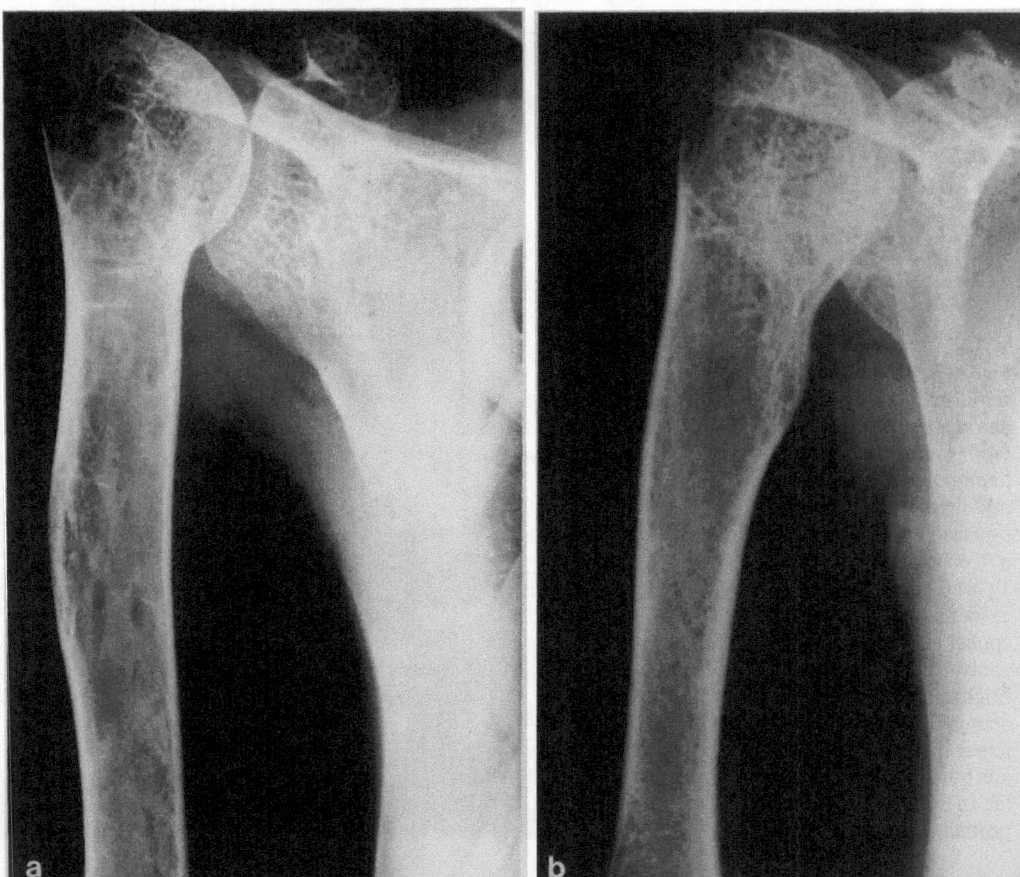

26 a, b

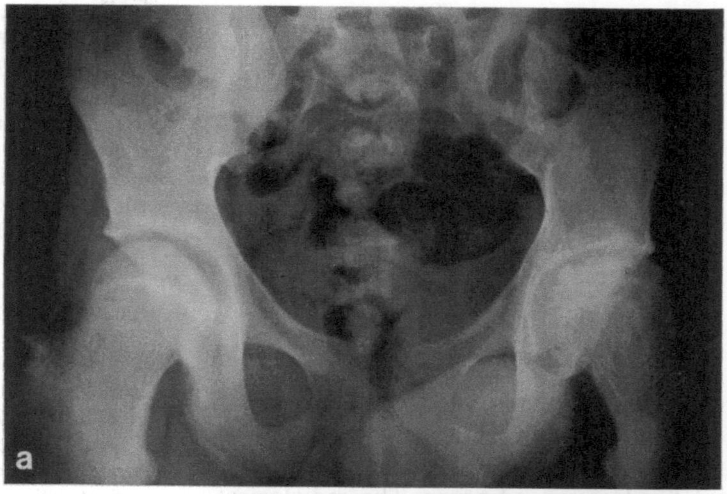

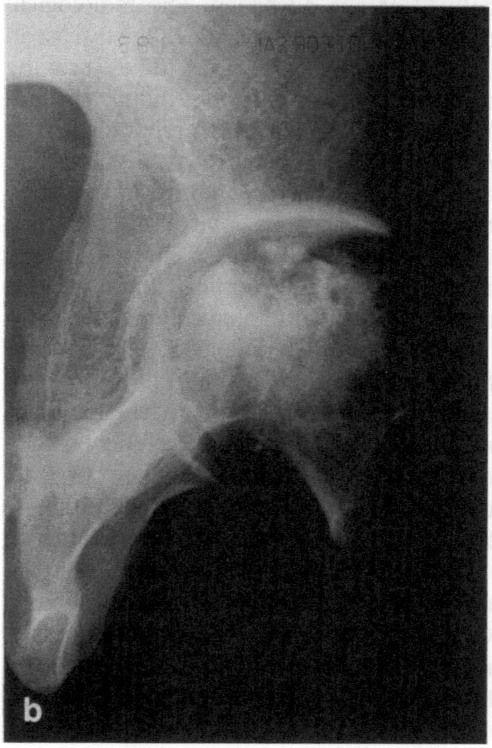

Fig. 28 a, b. Hip joint in thalassemia major: Legg-Calve-Perthes disease in two different patients (aseptic necrosis). There is deformity and flattening of the left femoral heads, associated with fragmenta

Fig. 25. Ribs in thalassemia major. The inferior margins of certain ribs upper left are indistinct and show cortical erosions. Note that the erosions occurred in ribs which are not particularly widened

Fig. 26 a, b. Humerus in two different patients with thalassemia major. There is deformity in both humeri and medial tilting of the proximal epiphyses due to premature fusion of the medial aspect of the epiphyseal line. There are also a few scattered lucencies

Fig. 27. Femur in thalassemia major. Partial premature fusion involving the posterior aspect of the epiphyseal line of the distal femur causes some tilting of the epiphysis posteriorly

cal radiolucent zones associated with flattening of the femoral head (Fig. 28 a,b). At a later stage, the X-ray findings are those of subluxation, flattening, and deformity of the femoral head [19, 29]. Orzincolo et al. [29] assumed that predisposing factors for this femoral abnomality were probably anemic hypoxia and/or osteopenia.

Summary

The skeletal changes in thalassemia major are radiologically indistinct during the 1st year of life, but they become more clearly defined as age advances. The radiological bone findings are diagnostic of the disease in long-standing severe cases. They are the result of marrow hypertrophy induced by prolonged and excessive hemopoiesis. As a result of the marked marrow hyperplasia and the increase in marrow volume, there is thinning of the cancellous bone of the entire skeleton system, as well as a rarefaction and absorbtion of the cortical bone readily demonstrable by radiological means.

The earliest radiological changes are found in small tubular bones of infants and children, particularly in the metacarpals and metatarsals. Skull changes, e.g., thickening of the diploë and vertical striation, are characteristic of thalassemia major, but they are manifested at a relatively advanced stage. They do not always run parallel to the changes in the rest of the skeleton or to the degree of anemia. Changes in the long tubular bones, spine, ribs, and phalanges have also been described, but they are less frequent and constitute less distinctive X-ray findings.

References

1. Andreou J, Gouliamos A, Kalovidouris A, Papailiou J, Papavasiliou C (1984) Bone marrow hyperplasia of the maxillary sinuses in β-thalassemia. J Comput Assist Tomogr 8: 180
2. Baker DA (1964) Roentgen manifestation of Cooley's anemia, Ann. NY Acad Sci 119: 641-661
3. Barlow RE, Goldman ML (1970) Computed tomography of the skeletal system. Comput Tomogr 2: 27–35
4. Boone ML, Swenson BE, Felson B (1964) Rib notching: its many causes. AJR 91: 1075–1088
5. Caffey J (1951) Cooley's erythroblastic anemia: some skeletal findings in adolescents and young adults. AJR 65: 547–560
6. Caffey J (1973) Pediatric x-ray diagnosis. Year Book Medical, Chicago
7. Caffey J (1957) Cooley's anemia: review of the roentgenographic findings in the skeleton. AJR 78: 381–391
8. Caffey TJ (1968) Anatomy, physiology and pathology of the blood supply of bones. J Bone Joint Surg 50: 766–783
9. Cassady JR, Berdon WE, Baker DH (1967) The "typical" spine changes of sickle-cell anemia in a patient with thalassemia major (Cooley's anemia). Radiology 89: 1065–1068
10. Cohen DM, Klatte CE, Baehner R, Smith J et al. (1984) Magnetic resonance imaging of bone marrow diseases in children. Radiology 151: 715–718
11. Cooley TB, Witwer ER, Lee R (1927) Anemia in children with splenomegaly and peculiar changes in bones, report of cases. Am J Dis Child 34: 347–363
12. Cravelle IH (1976) Clinical applications of xeroradiography. Br J Radiol 43: 557
13. Currarino G and Erlanson EM (1964) Premature fusion of epiphyses in Cooley's anemia. Radiology 83: 656–664
14. Danza F, Falappa P et al. (1982) Extramedullary hematopoiesis. AJR 139: 837–838
15. Drexler CJ, Stewart JR, Kincaid OW (1984) Diagnostic implication of rib notching. AJR 91: 1064–1074
16. Epstein SB (1962) The spine. Lea and Febiger. Philadelphia, pp 587–589
17. Feingold BF, Case JT (1963) Roentgenologic skull changes in anemias of childhood. AJR 29: 194–202
18. Fink IJ, Pastakia B, Barranger JA (1984) Enlarged phalangeal nutrient foramina in Gaucher disease and β-thalassemia. AJR 143: 647–949
19. Greenfield B, George (1986) Radiology of bone diseases, 4th edn. Lippincott, Philadelphia
20. Kaplan RI, Werther R, Castano FA (1964) Dental and oral findings in Cooley's anemia: a study of fifty cases. Ann NY Acad Sci 119: 664–666
21. Korsten J, Grossman H, Winchester Ph, et al. (1970) Extramedullary hematopoiesis in patients with thalassemia anemia. Radiology 95: 257–263
22. Lawson JP, Ablow RC, Pearson HA (1981) The ribs in thalassemia. Radiology 140: 663–679
23. Lawson JP, Ablow RC, Pearson HA (1983) Premature fusion of the proximal humeral epiphyses in thalassemia. AJR 140: 239–344

24. Lawson JP, Ablow RC, Pearson HA (1984) Calvarial and phalangeal vascular impressions in thalassemia. AJR 143: 641-645
25. Lee TJ, Sagel SS, Stanley JR (1983) Computed body tomography. Raven, New York
26. Moon LK, Genant KH, Helms AC, Chafetz IN et al. (1983) Musculoskeletal applications of nuclear magnetic resonance. Radiology 147: 161-171
27. Moseley JE (1963) Bone changes in hematologic disorders (roentgen aspects). Grune and Stratton, New York
28. Moseley JE (1975) Skeletal changes in the anemias. Semin Roentgenol 9: 169-184
29. Orzincolo C, Castaldi G, Scutellari PN et al. (1986) Aseptic necrosis of femoral head complicating thalassemia. Skeletal Radiol 15: 541-544
30. Papavasiliou C, Konstantopoulakis M, Priovolos J et al. (1979) The anterior costal margin mass in thalassemia major. Clin Radiol 30: 521-524
31. Papavasiliou C, Gouliamos A, Andreou J (1986) The marrow heterotopia in thalassemia. Eur J Radiol 6: 92-96
32. Pendergrass E, Schaeffer J, Hodes P (1956) The head the neck in roentgen diagnosis. Thomas, Springfield, pp 332-340
33. Scutellari P, Franceschini C, Orzincolo C (1981) Skeletal changes in treated β-thalassemia: a reappraisal. Rays (Roma) 7: 13-25
34. Scutellari PN, Orzincolo C, Tamarozzi R (1985) Xeroradiography in β-thalassemia, Skeletal Radiol 13: 39-43
35. Spencer JD (1979) Imaging factors for xeroradiography of the extremities. Br J Radiol 52: 51-55
36. Sutton D (1987) A textbook of radiology and imaging, 4th edn. Churchill Livingstone, Edinburgh

5 Osseous X-Ray Findings in Thalassemia Minor

P. Sfikakis

Introduction

The striking roentgenographic changes in the skeletal system encountered in homozygous thalassemia, particularly in thalassemia major, have been recognized for many years and are well documented in this book. However, little attention has been directed to the underlying osseous abnormalities of the carriers of thalassemia. Therefore, this chapter will deal with bone radiology of thalassemia trait or minor, on the basis of personal experience and the data so far reported on this subject in the literature.

In order to accomplish this task, it is necessary to define the terminology and clinical picture of the condition and to consider, as well, the most common circumstances under which a diagnosis can be obtained. Thalassemia trait represents heterozygous thalassemia in its more common and more benign state. It is a frequent condition in certain areas and is found especially in the Mediterranean populations with a frequency as high as 10% of the general population [19]. The carriers of the trait are not infrequently discovered accidentally; thus, examination for unrelated symptoms or investigation of a moderate anemia, palpable spleen, or family history are the more common causes of discovery of thalassemia trait.In addition to these causes, the discovery of silent bone rarefaction, always located at some part(s) of the skeleton, should be considered as a finding that can lead to recognition of thalassemia trait. In all such cases, there must be subsequent confirmation by suitable hematologic and biochemical screening tests, including hemoglobin (Hb) electrophoresis. Moreover bone rarefaction, if found, should not be attributed to other causes which may give osteopenia, mainly chronic anemia of other origin or the vulnerable effect of aging and sex upon bone matrix. Both situations may give rise to confusion in the interpretation of bone roentgenograms.

Radiographic Findings

The study of relatives of patients suffering from severe thalassemia drew attention to the possibility of observing bone changes in individuals with thalassemia trait. Thus, Caminopetros in 1938 [5] seems to have been the first to attach diagnostic value to X-ray findings of bones of trait carriers. He considered both osteoporosis and the hairbrush appearance of the calvarium to be rather frequent.

Subsequently, other authors studying healthy parents or siblings carrying the trait came to similar conclusions. Thus, Chini et al. [7] and Nicotra [11] added osteoporosis of the long bones as a usual diagnostic finding. Wintrobe et al. [20] described increased osteoporosis and thinning of the cortex of the long bones in a healthy trait carrier. Along the same lines, Smith [16] described a trabeculated zone of osteoporosis at the proximal portion of the right ulna in another carrier of the trait. Later, the same author [11] summarized his findings based on the study of members of 16 families; in some trait carriers of these families, a slightly enlarged diploic space, which finally appeared granular or mottled, was observed on lateral X-ray films of the skull. Castano et al. [6] reported osteoporosis of the frontal and parietal bones in a single subject with thalassemia trait. Daland and

Strauss [8] have presented a thesis establishing the value of mild X-ray changes of the skull as an additional criterion for diagnosis of thalassemia trait, whereas Silvestroni [14] and Astaldi and Tolentino [2] considered osteoporosis of the calvarium as the main change occurring in the thalassemia trait.

On the contrary, Kyhos and Corwin [9] did not confirm the existence of skull changes in a X-ray study of six adult carriers of the trait. Atkinson [4] did not observe bone changes in a roentgenographic study of the parents and relatives of two patients with thalassemia major.

This brief review of the literature reveals that description of X-ray bone findings in carriers of the trait was frequently based on single case reports or on rather incidental observations made during clinical studies on families. Such isolated data are rather insufficient and lack detail; furthermore, they are contradictory. Therefore, neither the incidence of osseous changes among a population of trait carriers nor their exact X-ray appearance could be estimated on the basis of these reports.

Sfikakis and Stamatoyannopoulos [18] carried out a controlled, prospective radiological appraisal of the bones and joints of 55 Greek carriers of the trait. The high incidence (7,4%) of thalassemia trait in young, otherwise healthy Greek individuals reported by Malamos et al. [10] provided the basis for their study. The trait carriers of this study were all clinically healthy males aged 18–25 years, and they all continued their habitual daily activities during the study. Intermediate thalassemia or microdrepanocytic disease, which are not rare conditions in Greece and are not infrequently diagnosed by chance, were ruled out by a relevant laboratory and clinical study of all individuals.

Roentgenographic surveys of each of the 55 carriers included a lateral projection of the skull, the lumbar spine, and the ribs. In 17 of these cases, an additional film was taken of the elbow (right or left). The interpretation of the radiographs was conducted in such a way as to rule out, or at least to minimize, subjective factors, as described previously [18]. Similar roentgenograms from 30 normal individuals matched for age, sex, and weight, taken under the same technical conditions, served as controls.

Table 1. Occurence and distribution of roentgenographic bone changes in 55 carriers of thalassemia trait [18].

	No. of cases
Carriers with bone changes	29
Skull changes, alone	17
Lumbar spine changes, alone	5
Elbow bone changes, alone[a]	2
Skull and lumbar spine changes, combined	3
Skull and elbow changes, combined	0
Lumbar spine and elbow changes, combined	1
Elbow and lumbar spine changes, combined	1
Carriers without bone changes	26

[a] X-ray films of the elbow were taken in 17 of the 55 carriers of the trait

The X-ray bone changes were analyzed as follows. In the skull, bone density in general, and particularly that of the diploic space, was appraised as were the width of the calvarium and appearance of inner and outer tables; a possible hairbrush appearance was also considered. In other bones, the structure was studied, including the appearance of the spongiosa and cortex, as well as of the distal parts of the long bones whenever a film of the elbow was available.

Osseous changes of varying degrees and distributions were observed on the X-ray films of 29 (53%) of the carriers studied. The remaining 26 (47%) carriers had normal roentgenograms. Table 1 summarizes the occurrence and distribution of the bone changes observed. Interestingly, changes in the ribs were not observed in any carriers.

Skull

In the skull, evident abnormalities concerned the diploë in 20 of the 55 carriers examined. These led to a hairbrush appearance of the skull, although they were less pronounced than those in the major form of thalassemia and were always circumscribed to one region

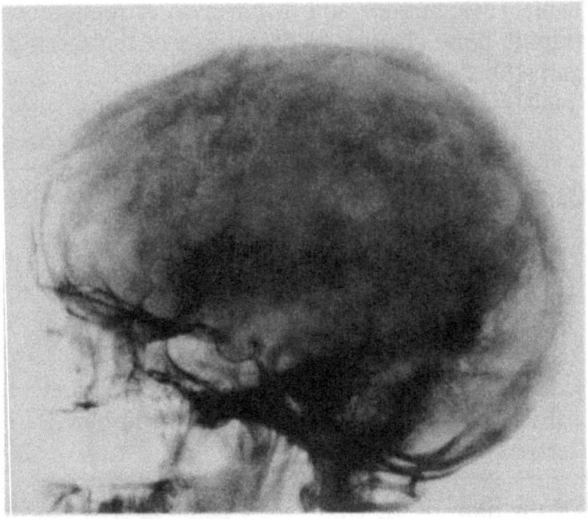

Fig. 1. Enlarged diploic space with hair-on-end apearance of the outer table in an asymptomatic male carrier of thalassemia

of the clavarium. In a few instances, this finding was more easily detectable by use of a hand lens. Abnormalities in the width of the diploë were evident in several cases. Figure 1 shows the roentgenogram of a healthy 23-year-old trait carrier presenting an abnormally enlarged diploë. In a few instances, there was a rarefying roentgenographic appearance of the diploic space, as well as abnormalities concerning the width of the tables. Such alterations were usually limited to the parietal region of the calvarium and/or to the surrounding parts of the frontal and occipital bones. Changes in the width of the tables and the diploic space were not classified in view of the wide variations known to occur normally.

A varying degree of hairbrush skull was noticed in all 20 carriers presenting an abnormal diploë. None had a hairbrush appearance troughout the calvarium such as is usually seen in thalassemia major. In ten subjects, the hair-on-end appearance concerned the outer table only; in seven, the vertical striation was confined to the diploic space; and in four trait carriers, the distinct trabeculae ran troughout the diploic space, from the inner to the outer table.

In our series, the site of the hairbrush appearance in the skull was as follows. In 2 subjects, the parietal bones and the neighboring part of the occipital bones were affected (Fig. 2); in 19 subjects, the hairbrush appearance was limited to the parietal bones: in 4 of these 19 subjects, this appearance extended throughout the parietal bone; in 4 subjects, the process was limited to the anterior third of the parietal bone, neighboring the frontal region; in 9 trait carriers, the same process was prominent in the middle third; and in remaining 2, the hairbrush appearance was noted posteriorly, near the occipital bones.

Among the 30 normal controls, a hairbrush appearance was recorded in only 3, as opposed to 20, of 55 carriers of thalassemia trait. It concerned only the outer table, and it was limited to the anterior and/or middle third of the parietal bone.

The striated appearance throughout the skull seen in advanced forms of hemolytic anemias was not observed in our series. In all cases, the cranial sinuses appeared normal, and overgrowth of the upper maxilla with expansion of its alveolar ridge was not observed on the lateral skull films. This was in agreement with the normal clinical appearance of the face and head of the carriers.

Lumbar Spine

The roentgenogram was normal in 45 of 55 cases. Of the remaining ten subjects – those with changes in the lumbar spine, with or without changes in other parts of the skeleton (Table 1) – nine showed a moderate porotic appearance of their lumbar spine, especially of L_4 and L_5, and one had a more diffuse osteoporosis throughout all lumbar vertebrae. However, heavy, irregular, and distorted trabeculae were never observed in the lumbar spine radiographs. None of the normal controls presented any abnormality of the lumbar spine.

Other Bones

All films revealed normal shape, structure and contours of the ribs; in particular, there was no broadening of the ribs. Lamellation of the inner layers of the ribs and irregular, distorted, or cystlike spaces were not observed in

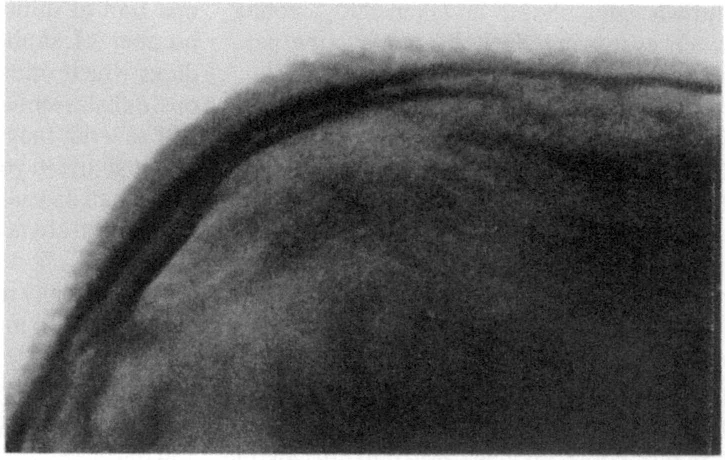

Fig. 2. Hairbrush appearance of the skull is more evident in the parietal bones

the roentgenograms, even using a hand lens. X-ray films of the elbow were taken at random in 17 of the 55 carriers examined. Thirteen subjects had a normal roentgenogram. The remaining four carriers, with or without X-ray changes of other bones, showed some degree of rarefaction involving the lower part of the humerus (Table 1). In one of these patients, the osteoporotic process, although mild, was also evident in the upper part of the ulna (Fig.3). No horizontal striations were observed near the ends of the diaphyses of the elbow bones, and the cortex was not thinned. The contours of the elbow bones were normal.

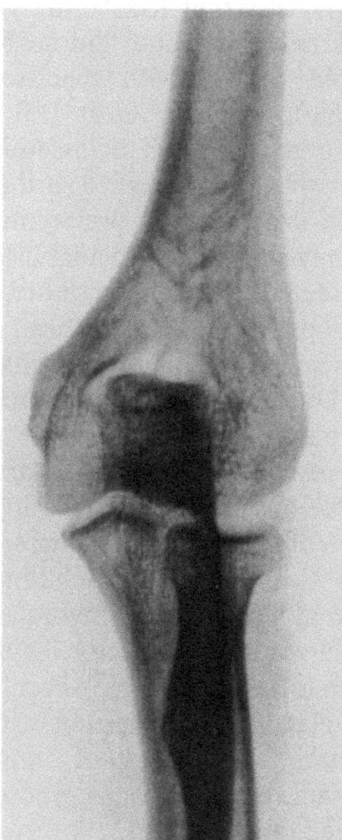

Fig. 3. Osseous rarefaction and horizontal striation of the humerus in an asymptomatic male with thalassemia trait. The upper part of the ulna is also osteoporotic

Conclusions

As a result of our studies, we came to the conclusion that osseous X-ray changes do occur in thalassemia minor. The skull is the part of the skeleton most often affected: 38% of the carriers seem to have X-ray modifications in the skull. The bones of the elbow and those of the lumbar spine are less frequently modified, i.e., in 23% and 18% of the carriers respectively. The ribs are unaffected. In other words, rarefying modifications of the humerus seem to be the most frequent abnormality next to those of the skull, while the lumbar spine presents bone rarefaction less frequently. The practical meaning of these findings is that osteoporosis of the humerus and lumbar spine should be taken into account when evaluating X-ray films of young persons of Mediterranean origin.

The pathogenesis of osseous rarefaction in thalassemia minor carriers is the same as that in thalassemia major. It may be attributed to normoblastic hyperplasia, although this is much less evident than in overt thalassemia syndromes [2, 19]. However, other constitutional factors concerning the structure of the bone itself may be operating in the pathogenesis of osseous rarefaction. Such factors, perhaps genetic in origin and not necessarily present in all trait carriers, may explain why osseous X-ray changes are not present in every case of thalassemia minor.

As far as the possible occurrence of arthritis in thalassemia minor is concerned, the literature is poor, and the data so far reported cannot be considered as definite or conclusive. Thus, Abou Rizk et al. [1] described aseptic necrosis of both femoral heads in a 28-year-old female with thalassemia minor (AA_2Hb). Schlumpf et al. [13] described a series of patients with thalassemia minor and nonerosive, seronegative arthritis of the middle-sized joints preferentially. X-ray study revealed juxta-articular osteoporosis of the affected joints; furthermore, one patient had aseptic necrosis of the head of humerus. It was suggested that the mechanism of the latter bone lesion is long-standing medullary hyperplasia, with the possible presence of bone marrow fat emboli and an increase in intraosseous pressure. Discussing the combination of arthritis and thalassemia minor, Abou Rizk et al. [1] and Schlumpf et al. [13], state that long-standing medullary hyperplasia is a contributing factor for the synovitis seen in these patients. However, the possibility of classifying the carriers with "arthritis" within the framework of "nondisease", a newly accepted rheumatic syndrome, cannot be ruled out.

Summary

The occurrence, nature, and other parameters of osseous X-ray involvement in thalassemia trait or minor have been explored in a number of studies. Roentgenographic findings which mimic those seen in homozygous β-thalassemia do exist. Their incidence and severity may depend on the population under study: in young adult carriers aged not more than 25 years, abnormal X-ray findings can be seen at a rate of up to 53%. The changes consist of bone rarefaction of varying degrees, usually mild, located at some part(s) of the skeleton most often the skull, and less frequently in the elbow and lumbar spine. Aseptic necrosis of the femoral head has been reproted in the literature very sporadically, and the possibility of change coexistence cannot be excluded. The pathogenesis of the osseous lesions may be attributed to normoblastic hyperplasia present in the bone marrow of trait carriers, although to a lesser extent than in thalassemia major patients.

The possibility that one is dealing with some of the many forms of intermediate thalassemia or of microdrepanocytic disease, rhater than with cases of simple thalassemia minor, should be ruled out when facing conditions characterized by a very mild symptomatology and X-ray findings such as are described in this review; such conditions are not rare in certain populations.

References

1. Abou Rizk MN, FW Nasr, RA Frayha (1977) Aseptic necrosis in thalassemia minor. Arthritis Rheum 20: 1147
2. Astaldi G, Tolentino P (1952) Physiopathologie et clinique de la thalassémie. Sang 23: 453
3. Astaldi G, Tolentino PE, Sacchetti C (1951) La Talassemia. Tipographia del libro, Pavia
4. Atkinson DW (1939) Erythroblastic anemia: report of two cases in adult siblings. Am J Med Sci 198: 376
5. Caminopetros J (1938) Recherches sur l'anémie érythroblastique infantile des peuples de la Méditerranée orientale. Ann Med Int. (Paris) 43: 104
6. Castano M, Papachristos G, Juili H (1954) Les images osseuses de la thalassémie ou anémie de Cooley à propos d'une observation familiale. J Radiol Electrol 35: 465
7. Chini V, Ferannini AE, Pona G (1939) Indagini sulla familiarita dell' anemia mediterranea a morbo di Cooley. Minerva Med 30: 377

8. Daland GA, Strauss MB (1948) The genetic relation and clinical differentiation of Cooley's trait. Blood, 3: 438
9. Kyhos ED, Corwin VM (1957) Mediterranean anaemia trait in adults. J Am Med Assoc 12: 335
10. Malamos B, Fessas PH, Stamatoyannopoulos G (1962) Types of thalassemia trait carriers as revealed by a study of their incidence in Greece. Br J Haematol 8: 5
11. Nicotra A (1939) Indagini sulla familiarita dell' anemia mediterranea. Radiol Med (Torino) 26: 720
12. Schlumpf U (1978) Thalassemia minor and aseptic necrosis, a coincidence? Arthritis Rheum 21: 280
13. Schlumpf U, Gerber N, Bünzli H, Elsässer U, Pestalozzi A, Böni A (1977) Arthritiden bei Thalassemia minor. Schweiz Med Wochenschr 107: 1156
14. Silverstroni E (1949) Microcitemia e malattie a substrato microcitemico. 50th Congress Soc Ital Med Interna, Rome
15. Smith CH (1942) Mediterranean (Cooley's) anaemia in a young of nineteen years observed since early childhood. J Pediatr 20: 270
16. Smith CH (1943) Familial blood studies in cases of Mediterranean (Cooley's) anaemia. Am J Dis Child 65: 681
17. Snapper I (1957) Bone diseases in medical practice, vol I. Grune and Stratton, New York
18. Sfikakis P, Stamatoyannopoulos G (1963) Bone changes in thalassemia trait. An X-ray appraisal of 55 cases. Acta Haematol (Basel) 29: 193
19. Wintrobe MM (1974) Clinical hematology, 7th edn.Lea and Febiger, Philadelphia
20. Wintrobe MM, Matthews E, Pollack R, Dobyns BA (1940) A familial hemopoietic disorder in Italian adolescents and adults. J Am Med Assoc 114: 1530

6 A Reappraisal of Some Skeletal Changes in Currently Treated β-Thalassemia

P.N. Scutellari, F. Franceschini, and C. Orzincolo

Introduction

It is common knowledge that in β-thalassemic syndromes bone alterations are absent at birth, but may be appreciated radiologicallly after the 1st year of life and become characteristic during early childhood [3, 4, 10, 11, 41, 52, 55, 73, 82]. Bone marrow hyperplasia is generally considered responsible for skeletal changes [12, 14, 18, 27, 30, 50, 77] (osteopenia with widening of the medulla, thinning of the cortex in long bones and reactive periosteal new bone formation). These alterations, described by Cooley and Lee in 1925, are diagnostic and characteristic in the severe forms of anemia (homozygous β-thalassemia). They involve the entire skeleton but are usually more conspicuous in the skull and extremities [4, 10, 11, 41, 52, 53, 55]. With advancing age, skeletal lesions disappear in the peripheral segments, where red marrow is converted into yellow marrow, but they persist in the axial skeleton, where the bone marrow remains red. Therefore, in adolescence and early adulthood bone changes are particularly common in the skull, pelvis, and spine. Pseudotumors of extramedullary hematopoiesis may occur in paravertebral sites and in many other organs and tissues [8, 22, 45, 57, 58]. This process is far more frequent in thalassemia intermedia [13, 66].

Presently, treatment of β-thalassemia [47, 49, 76–79] depends on the following three basic supports: (a) repeated blood transfusions to treat anemia [80, 81] and to prevent cardiac dysfunction and failure [60], (b) chelation therapy to alleviate the iron overload resulting from transfusions [6, 28, 64] and (c) psychological advice to patients an their relatives [76]. Splenectonomy is recommended when hypersplenism develops (20, 63). Recently, marrow transplantation has been attempted [46].

Until 1965, thalassemic patients were transfused infrequently, with hemoglobin (Hb) levels of 5–6 g/100 ml, i.e. low-transfusion regimen [47, 49]. Modern therapeutic management of thalassemia major has changed the course of the disease and the spectrum of many radiological manifestations [67–69, 72]. Patients are maintained at a higher baseline level of Hb (above 8 g/100 ml). They are generally in better health and have smaller organs (e.g., liver and heart). Body growth, particularly height and weigth, is fairly satisfactory. Survival time is markedly prolonged, and these patients go on to adult life and may even procreate. Skeletal lesions that appear later are less severe and localized in the axial region [50]. Radiological changes are explained on the basis of the relationship between the proliferating marrow and the surrounding bone; therefore, bone abnormalities depend on the type of transfusion regimen. The hypertransfusion regimen, begun early in life, will prevent development of lesions: many of the "typical" features of thalassemia do not appear in early childhood, and most of the clinical problems that occur after the 1st decade are the result of iron accumulation following blood transfusions [17]. On the other hand, in the majority of cases abnormal radiological findings do not regress with a low-transfusion regimen [7, 61, 65].

Synopsis of Current Skeletal Changes

Our present review had to overcome many obstacles in setting up a quantitative comparison between various groups of patients, who differ widely among themselves in both severity of anemia and involvement of individual organs, and whose treatments also differ significantly. Nevertheless, our data confirm that the most noticeable finding is the late appearance of bone lesions in most cases [68]. Their intensity and extension may be unremarkable as a result. Some peculiar "target" areas of the skeleton are less involved, in relation to regression of marrow hyperplasia. The disease is commonly evident in the 1st year of life. If an accurate diagnosis is made [16] at this stage, and a regular blood transfusion regimen is established, subsequent growth and development may be relatively normal, at least over the following decade [77].

Skull

In about 16% of our thalassemic patients [68] undergoing current treatment, deformities of the skull and facial bones are not present, and, by the time the subjects reach adulthood, the bones develop quite normally. This finding is particularly important because in a very large number of cases, the classical skeletal lesions of thalassemia are prevented and/or markedly modified in their aspect and degree by therapy, and they may dissapear completely after puberty.

On the other hand, the lesion most frequently observed in the first and subsequent radiographic investigations remains; widening of the diploic space with osteopenia and a mottled appearance. Nevertheless, swelling of the diploic space is not diffuse in the skull but is localized in the frontal area (helmeted aspect). Sometimes, the calvarium becomes hollow (camelback pattern); the occipital squamosa, inferior to the internal occipital protuberance, is not involved because of deficiency in marrow. Radial arrangement of the diploic space is present in 5%–18% of our cases. It is important to emphasize that in the hairbrush pattern of younger patients, the spiculae are always confined to the frontal and/or parietal bones, and they may disappear gradually, as the child grows, and with therapeutic management. However, with inadequately transfused thalassemic children, the incidence of vertical striae in the diploic space is much higher at first observation (22.5%) and increases progressively with advancing age. It is also noteworthy that the hair-on-end appearance is already diffuse in all the skull bones [68].

The thickness of the diploic space, measured on the lateral view of the skull, is markedly pronounced in the frontal area in children (mean, 11.9 mm), while in the parietal area the mean value is inferior (8.6 mm). With advancing age, the diploic space increases in thickness in conformity to the total growth of the skull, but these values are less conspicuous than those observed in the group of nontreated thalassemic patients [68].

Regression of thickness of the diploic space is less evident in patients who are known to have been affected by anemia only in childhood or who have been defectively transfused. Nevertheless, although the striated skull may disappear, entirely or partially, the homogeneous, mottled, spongy appearance remains, whereas in correctly treated patients, diploic thickness is minimal and sometimes falls within normal value ranges. Generally, it is limited to the frontal area at the beginning of the disease, with an elevated aspect (bossing of the skull).

The vascular impressions in the calvarium tend to appear normal in patients who have been transfused at an early age, whereas they are largest, tortuous, and widened in those who have never been transfused or have been on low-transfusion regimens [40].

Obliteration of the air spaces in the paranasal sinuses is minimal or absent in many cases. Overgrowth of facial bones, facial disfigurement, and grotesque appearance are rarely seen [44]. In a few cases, maxillary hypertrophy and malocclusion require surgical correction [36, 70, 74]. The term which

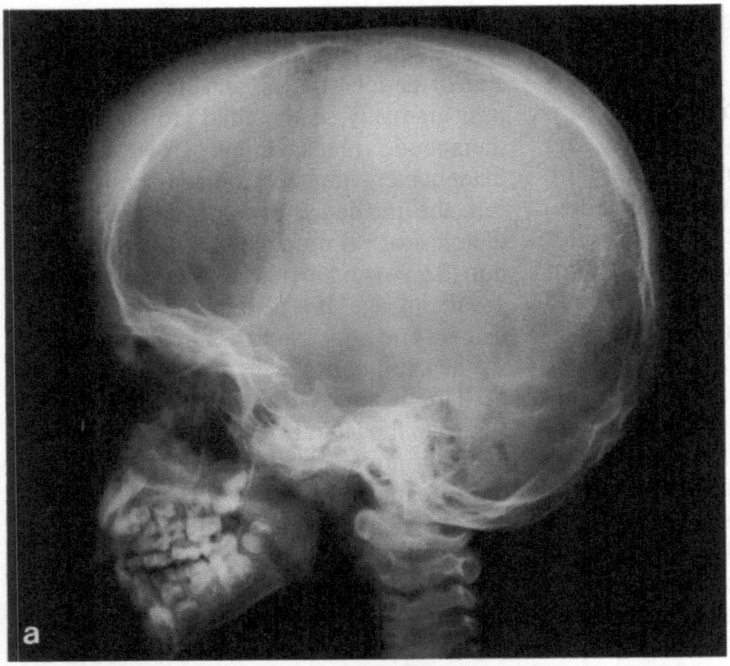

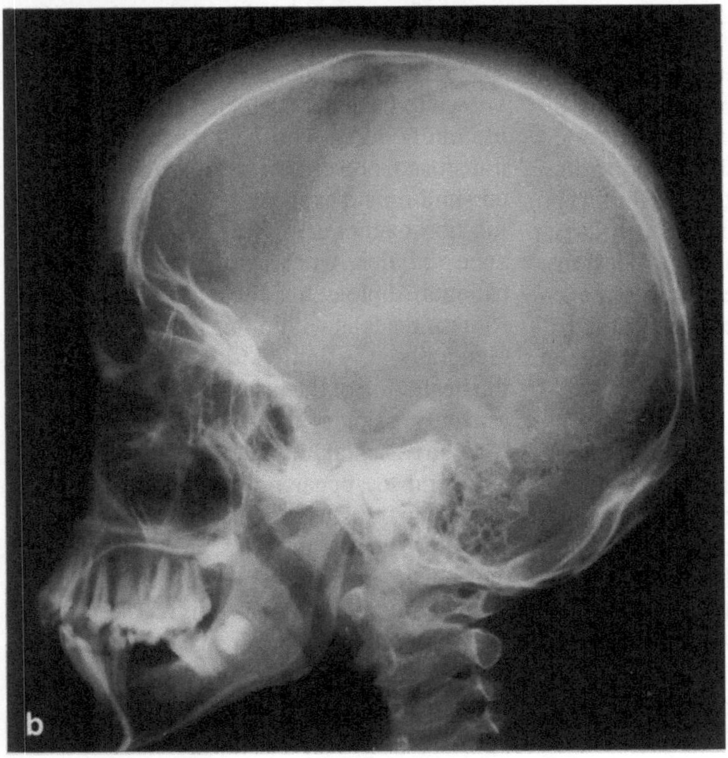

Fig. 1 a–c. Skull findings in correctly transfused thalassemic subjects. **a** Increased width of the diploic space, located mainly in the frontal area (bossing of the skull), with scattered vertical striae. **b** Harmonic width of the diploic space, with mottled, spongy appearance and atrophy of the outer table. **c** Camelback aspect in the outline of the calvarium, with evident radial striations in the thickened frontal and parietal bones

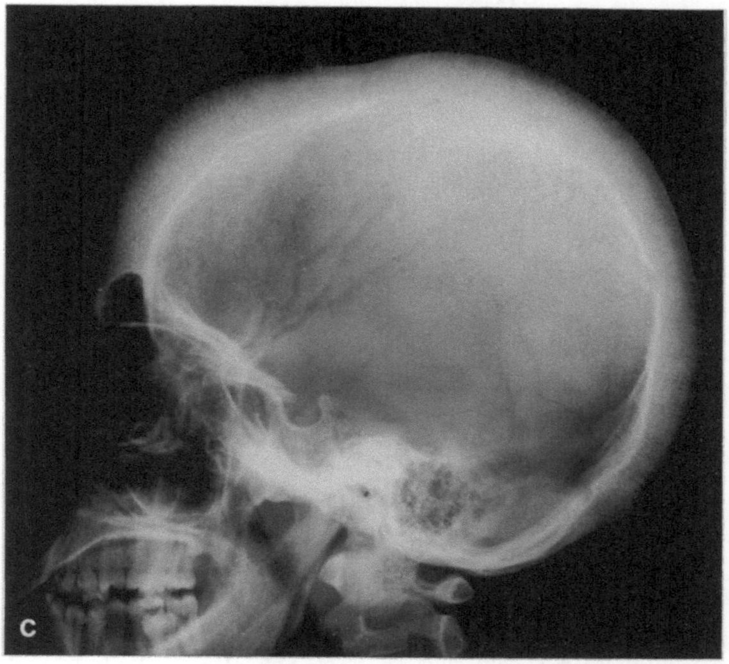

Fig. 1 c

best describes the facial abnormalities is now "rodent facies" [4, 62]. Swelling of facial bones is absent in the milder forms of the disease. The radiological findings of the skull are shown in Figs. 1 and 2.

Hand

The hand is usually involved in the early years of life and shows a characteristic rarefaction (Fig. 3). Its pattern suggests the presence of many small cysts ("wormeaten"), while the cortex on the shaft of the tubular bones is very thin, with a washed-out appearance [4, 11]. The medullary canal is wide and is crossed by the remaining coarsened trabeculae. Changes are most pronounced in the metacarpals and phalanges, in which inversion of the outline of the shaft is also present. Enlargement of the nutrient foramina of the phalanges has already been reported [31, 40]. When present, the foramina are circular, varying in size from less than 1 mm to more than 2 mm, and they are seen most often in the distal portion of the proximal or middle phanlanx. Usually, foramina are identified in more than two phalanges (Fig. 4).

With advancing age, and following current treatment, regression and eventual disappearance of the lesions are observed in almost all cases. Nevertheless, all thalassemic patients, particularly those undergoing incorrect treatment, show bone deficiency in metacarpal surfaces, with increased medullary diameter, sometimes associated with blurring of the trabeculae. The first metacarpal is clearly square, in patients correctly or incorrectly transfused, and remains so in adult life, when changes in the hand usually regress [68].

Quantitative radiographic measurements (e.g., cortical thickness, cortical area, and metacarpal bone mass) always remain inferior to those in healthy controls, particularly in patients not undergoing current treatment [68]. The amount of bone can be evaluated radiologically by computing the bone mass of the second left metacarpal [5]: the measurement of the outer diameter of the periosteal width (D), the inner diameter of the medullary space (d), and the combined cortical thickness (D–d) at the midpoint of the metacarpal shaft are generally used. The cortical area ($D^2 - d^2$) and the metacarpal bone mass [$(D^2-d^2)/D^2$] are then calculated [1].

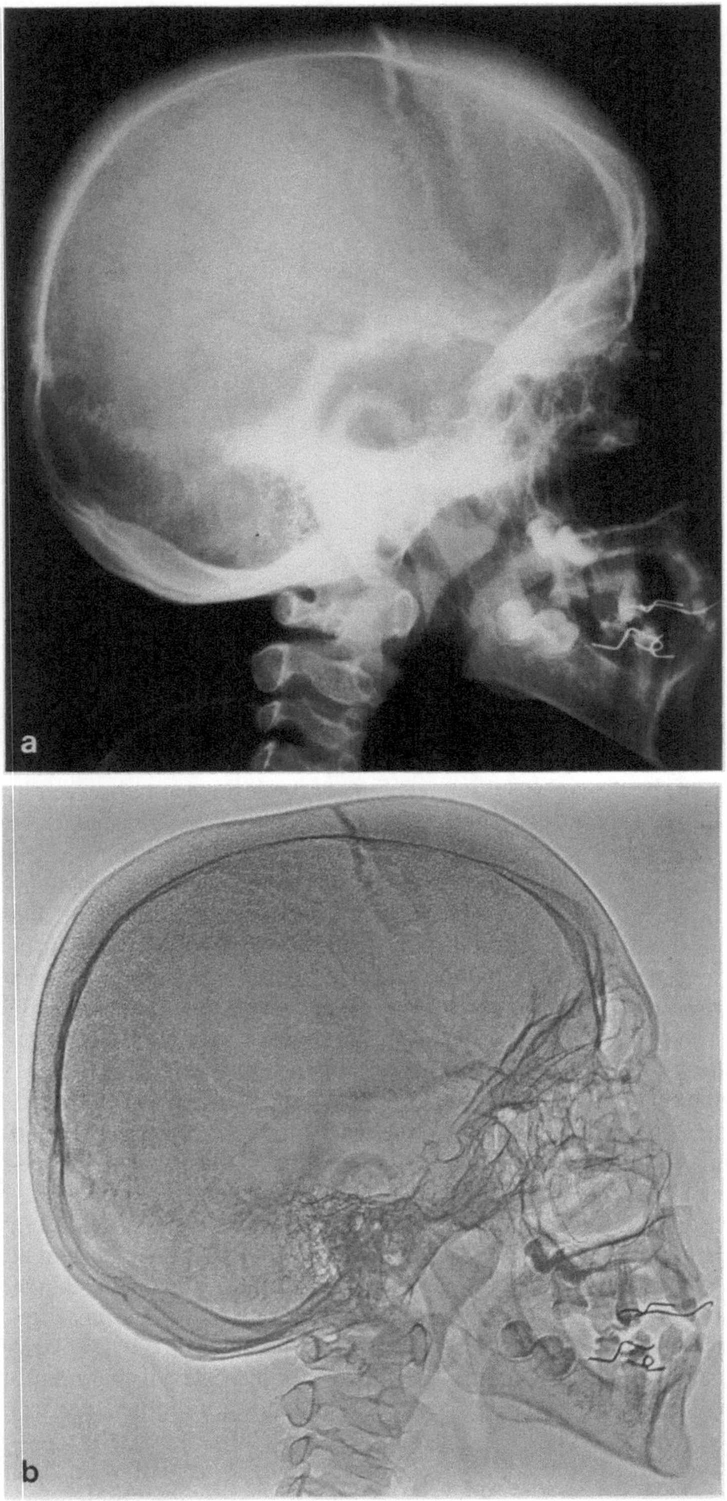

Fig. 2. **a** Radiograph and **b** xerography of the skull in an adequately treated 14-year-old male thalassemic. The diploic space, particularly the outer table, is better demonstrated in **b** than in **a** because of the specific edge contrast enhancement and wide recording latitude peculiar to the xerographic method

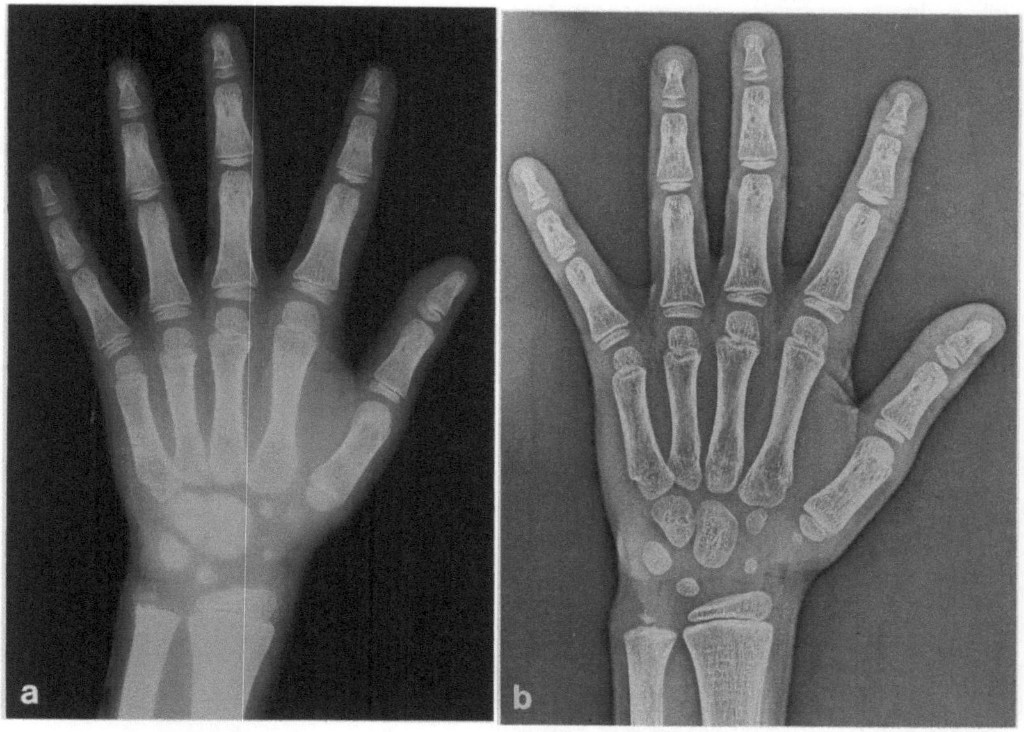

Fig. 3. a Radiograph and **b** xerograph of the hand in a 9-year-old male: osteopenia, cortical atrophy, and minor marrow expansion are present. Lesions are more clearly visible when the xerographic technique is used

These quantitative measurements are a simple and reproducible method to estimate bone mass indirectly, during ageing and in various pathologic conditions (e.g., hemolytic anemias). Unfortunately, there is a large variability in the amount of bone within one age and sex group, even in normal bone, which is related to skeletal size difference [23, 26, 29, 51]. Moreover, in thalassemia major the measurements of both the outer and inner margins of the cortical layer are particularly difficult to appreciate because of exaggerated thinning of cortical bone in the metacarpal shaft, due to widening of the medullary space [25, 68]. Nevertheless, these measurements have improved our knowledge of both the radiographic picture of the hand in anemic disorders and remodelling of bone mass. In thalassemic men and women, metacarpal bone mass is objectively and significantly reduced, as compared with normal controls. This reflects a severe loss of cortical thickness and cortical area and a conspicuous increase in width of the bone marrow cavity. Since osteopenia may be due to periosteal or endosteal resorption, it is obvious that in β-thalassemia the loss of bone mass is principally related to endosteal resorption [68]. Similar bone changes are observed in the foot (Fig. 5).

Ribs

A variety of rib changes have been noted in β-thalassemia, even in Cooley's original report [38, 39, 71]. The entire rib is usually widened: multiple involvements are far more pronounced posteriorly, but significant expansion of the anterior portion has also been reported [59] (Fig. 6). Osteopenia is widespread, with thinning of the cortex, and it is sometimes associated with localized lucent defects of bone density. Cortical erosions, which frequently occur in the inferior margin

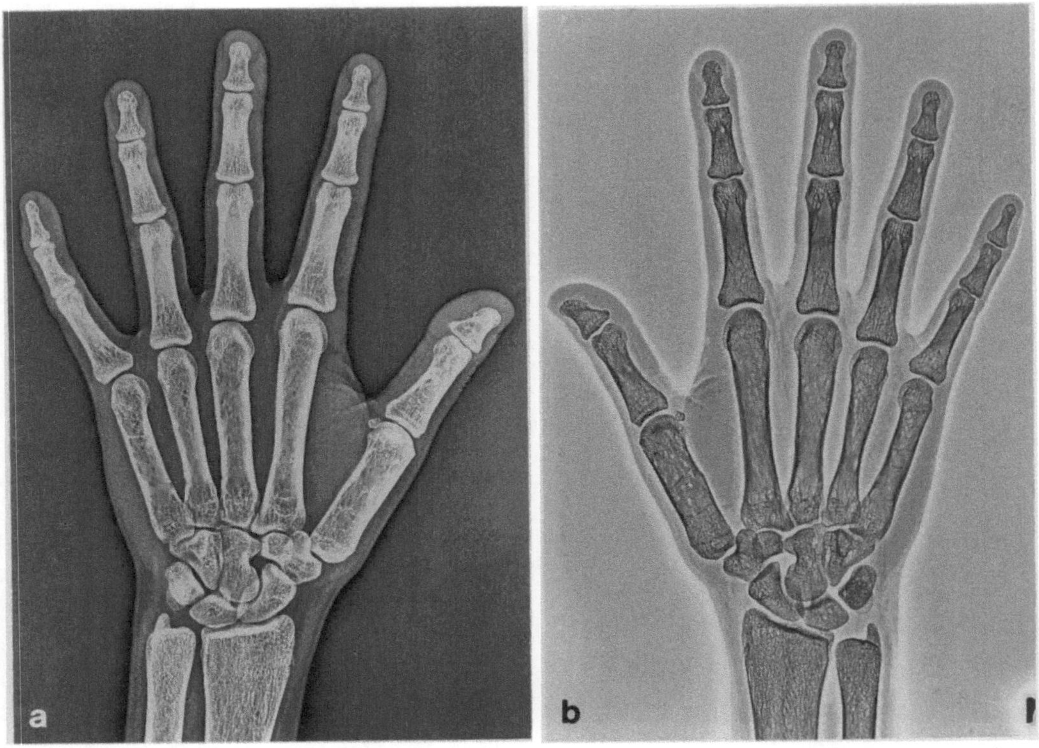

Fig. 4 a, b. Xerographs of the hand in a 20-year old female, developed in a negative (**a**) and positive (**b**) mode. Widening of medullary cavities and thinness of cortex in the shaft of long bones are well documented. Note regression of the classical cystlike appearance seen exclusively in severe forms of thalassemia major and enlargement of the nutrient foramina in the middle phalanges. The outline of the shaft of metacarpals and phalanges is quite normal. The metacarpal of the thumb is clearly and significantly square

of the ribs, are well defined and sharply marginated. Sometimes, they look like the notching produced by coarctation of the aorta. The "rib within a rib" consists of a line of increased density, localized in the central area of the rib and separated from the superior and inferior cortices by the medulla. It is particularly noticeable in the mid and anterior portions of the rib. This lesion is to be found only in thalassemic patients [38, 53]. A fine linear subcortical lucency is frequently seen parallel and close to the superior margin [38]. It is explained as a loss of the adjacent medullary trabeculae, provoked by marrow hyperplasia. This lesion is the abnormality that most commonly regresses, after adequate blood transfusions.

The development of rib findings is related to the patient's age at the time of transfusion therapy: hypertransfusion will only prevent the development of any rib abnormalities if it is begun early in life [39].

Additional Osseous Findings

In thalassemic children, a common change is premature fusion of the epiphyses in the tubular bones of the extremities, particularly in the proximal humerus (Fig. 7) and distal femur, resulting in deformity and shortening [21]. Furthermore, thalassemic patients have deficiencies in endocrine functions – related to an iron overload [14, 15, 32, 37] – and

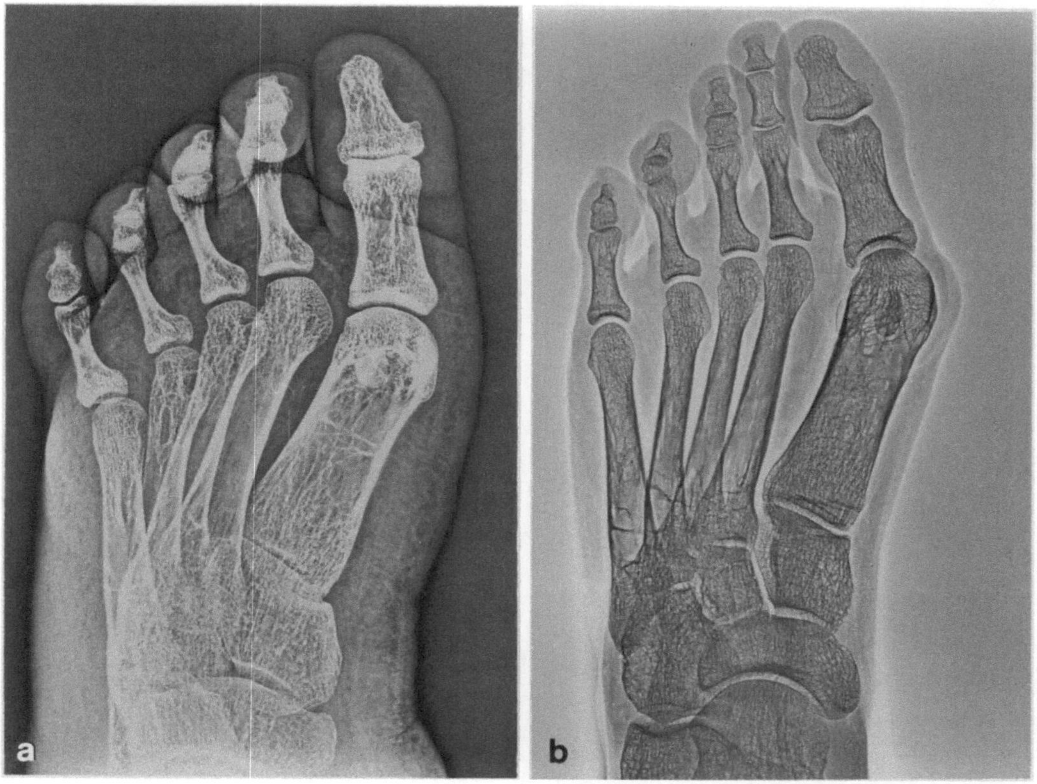

Fig. 5 a, b. Xerographs of the foot **a** in a 37-year-old male not currently being treated and **b** in an adequatly transfused 20-year-old female. The type and development of the lesions are the same as those observed in the hand. Note thinning of cortex in the tubular bones, with coarsened trabeculae across the medulla and multiple cystlike lesions within the distal portion of metatarsals

protein metabolism, which contribute to weakening of the bones.

Spontaneous fractures are frequent in long bones [24, 62, 75], which must be expected in view of severe osteopenia. Such fractures recur at the same site and heal relatively slowly [33, 62]. Recently [56], osteonecrosis of the femoral head has been reported as complicating thalassemia, also in transfused patients.

Summary

The age at which patients are first transfused will influence the type of abnormalities that develop [9, 49, 54, 78]. Today, skeletal findings of thalassemia major have changed their classical radiographic patterns [35, 44]. In the skull, the diploic space may become normal, overgrowth of facial bones is moderate [2], pneumatization of the paranasal sinuses is not completely impeded by swelling of the jaw, and the hairbrush pattern may disappear completely. The normalized aspect of the hand remains a typical site of differentiation between prepubertal patients and adults. The same changes are seen in the foot.

Nevertheless, in spite of modern therapy, an important retardation of both height and weight remains, causing dwarfism and infantilism [34, 42, 43, 48, 83]. In children over 10 years of age, a significant dissociation is also observed between the findings in the skull and axial skeleton and those in long bones, but it is less evident than in the past.

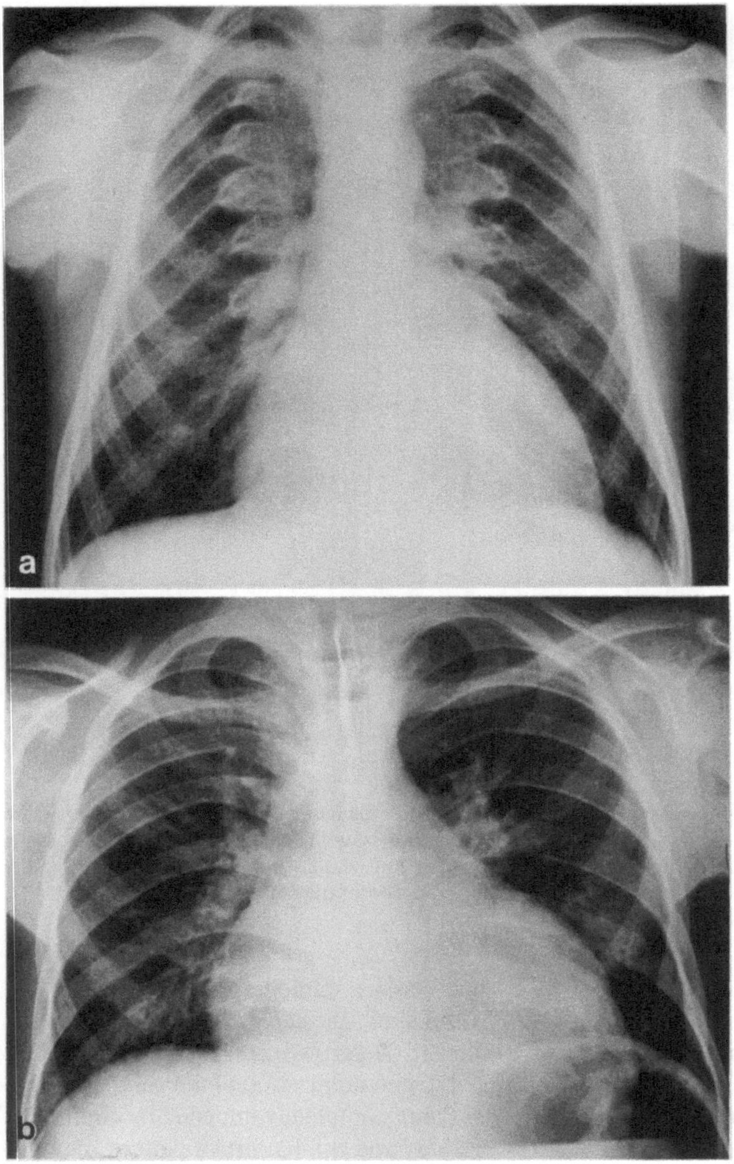

Fig. 6 a, b. Chest films. **a** In a nontreated thalassemic patient, widening of ribs, more pronounced in the posterior portion, and linear subcortical lucencies along the superior margin of the ribs, are present. **b** In a patient hypertransfused early, the ribs are completely normal

References

1. Andresen J, Nielsen HE (1986) Amount of bone and bone remodelling in normal subjects and in patients with chronic renal failure. Acta Radiol (Diagn) (Stockh) 27: 341–346
2. Asbell MB (1964) Orthodontic aspects of Cooley's anemia. Ann NY Acad Sci 119: 662–663
3. Astaldi G, Tolentino P, Sacchetti C (1951) La talassemia, Tipografia del Libro, Pavia
4. Baker DH (1964) Roentgen manifestations of Cooley's anemia. Ann NY Acad Sci 119: 641–661
5. Barnett E, Nordin BEC (1960) The radiological diagnosis of osteoporosis: a new approach. Clin Radiol 11: 166–174
6. Barry M, Flynn DM, Letsky EA, Risdon RA (1974) Long-term chelation therapy in thalassemia major: effect on liver iron concentration, iron histology and clinical progress. Br Med J 2: 16–25

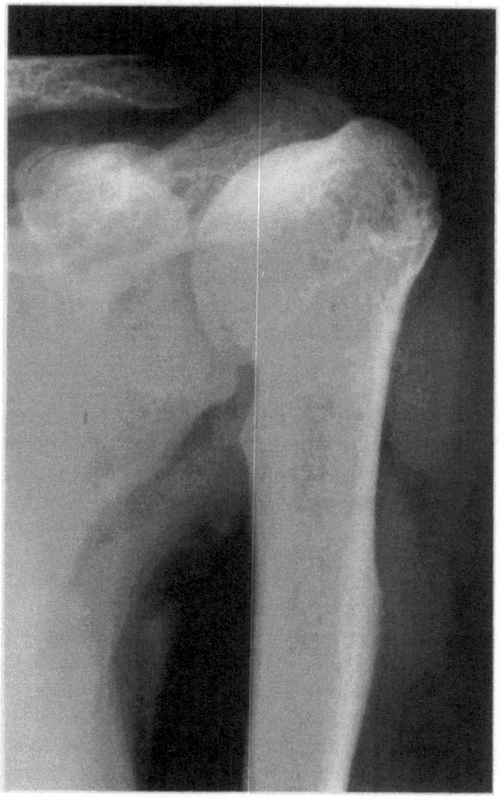

Fig. 7. Roentgenogram of the left shoulder in a 15-year-old male. There is premature fusion of the medial aspect of the proximal humeral epiphysis

7. Beard MEJ, Necheles TF, Allen DM (1969) Clinical experience with intensive transfusion therapy in Cooley's anemia. Ann NY Acad Sci 165: 415-422
8. Bron LJ, Paquelet JR, Tetalman MR (1980) Intrathoracic extramedullary hematopoiesis: appearance on 99m Tc sulfur colloid marrow scan. AJR 134: 1254-12255
9. Brook CGD, Thompson EN, Marshall WC, Whitehouse RH (1969) Growth in children with thalassemia major and effect of two different transfusion regimens. Arch Dis Child 44: 612-615
10. Caffey J (1951) Cooley's erythroblastic anemia. Some skeletal findings in adolescent and young adults. AJR 65: 547-560
11. Caffey J (1957) Cooley's anemia: a review of the roentgenographic findings in the skeleton. AJR 78: 381-391
12. Cajozzo A, Perricone R, Tolomeo M (1985) Le talassemie. Haematologica (Pavia) 70: 341-358
13. Camascella C, Saglio G, Pich PG, Canavoso P, Ferraris R, Bianco G, Mazza U (1981) Thoracic extramedullary hematopoiesis in thalassemia intermedia during adult life: a report of 9 cases. Haematologica (Pavia) 66: 613-626
14. Cammisa M, Sabella G (1967) Considerazioni clinico-radilogiche sulla patogenesi delle alterazioni ossee nella talassemia major. Nunt Radiol 33: 77-101
15. Canale VC, Steinherz P, New M, Erlandson M (1974) Endocrine function in thalassemia major. Ann NY Acad Sci 232: 333-345
16. Cao A, Rosatelli MC (1985) Diagnosi prenatale di emoglobinopatie ereditarie. Haematologica (Pavia) 70: 361-368
17. Caronia F, Mancuso L, Rigano P, Castellano S, Bondi F, Maggio A (1985) Danno d'organo da accumulo de ferro in pazienti talassemici. Haematologica (Pavia) 70: 383-390
18. Castaldi G (1986) Talassemie, In: Baserga A (ed) Ematologica clinica. UTET, Torino, pp 111-132
19. Costin G, Kogut MD, Hyman CB, Ortega JA (1979) Endocrine abnormalities in thalassemia major. Am J Dis Child 133: 497-502
20. Citarella P, Marco P, Pecorella M, Cajozzo A (1979) La splenectomia nella talassemia grave ed intermedia. Atti XXVI Congr Naz Soc Ital Ematol, Torino
21. Currarino G, Erlandson ME (1964) Premature fusion of epiphysis in Cooley's anemia. Radiology 83: 656-664
22. Danza FM, Falappa P, Leone G, Pincelli G (1982) Extramedullary hematopoiesis. AJR 139: 837-838
23. Dequeker J (1980) Measurement of bone mass and bone remodelling in vivo. Value of the radiogrammetric approach. Acta Rheumatol 4: 40-75
24. Diness DM, Canale VC, Arnold WD (1976) Fractures in thalassemia. J Bone Joint Surg (Am) 58: 662-666
25. Doxiadis S, Georgaki E, Papamichael D, Papadakou-Lagogianni S, Lapatsanis P (1978) Bone density in thalassemic children during the course of the disease. Pediat Res 12: 811-815
26. Evans RA, McDonnel GD, Schieb M (1978) Metacarpal cortical area as an index of bone mass. J. Radiol 51: 428-431
27. Fessas P, Loukopoulos D (1974) The β-thalassemias. Clin Haematol 3: 411-440
28. Fink H (1964) Transfusion hemochromatosis in Cooley's anemia. Ann NY Acad Sci 119: 680-685
29. Garn SM (1981) Contributions of the radiographic image to our knowledge of human growth. AJR 137: 231-239
30. Gabutti V, Piga A, Cordero A, Fortina P. Times F (1981) Erythropoiesis in thalassemia. Haematologica (Pavia) 66: 257-268

31. Fink IJ, Pastakia B, Barranger JA (1984) Enlarged phalangeal nutrient foramina in Gaucher disease and β-thalassemia major. AJR 143: 647-949
32. Flink DM, Fairney A, Jackson D, Clayton BE (1976) Hormonal changes in thalassemia major. Arch Dis Child 51: 828-836
33. Gratwick GM, Bullough PG, Bohne WH, Markenson AL, Peterson CM (1978) Thalassemic osteoarthropathy. Ann Intern Med 88: 494-501
34. Johnston FE, Krogman WM (1964) Patterns of growth in children with thalassemia major. Ann NY Acad Sci 119: 667-679
35. Johnston FE, Rosemann JM (1967) The effects of more frequent transfusions upon bone loss in thalassemia major. Pediat Res 1: 479-483
36. Kaplan RI, Werther R, Castano FA (1964) Dental and oral findings in Cooley's anemia: a study of fifty cases. Ann NY Acad Sci 119: 664-666
37. Lassman MN, O'Brien RT, Pearson HA, Wise JK, Donabedian RK, Felig P, Genel A (1974) Endocrine evaluation in thalassemia major. Ann NY Acad Sci 232: 226-237
38. Lawson JP, Ablow RC, Pearson HA (1981) The ribs in thalassemia. I. The relationship to therapy, Radiology 140: 663-672
39. Lawson JP, Ablow RC, Pearson HA (1981) The ribs in thalassemia. II. The pathogenesis of the changes. Radiology 140: 673-679
40. Lawson JP, Albow RC, Pearson HA (1984) Calvarial and phalangeal vascular impressions in thalassemia. AJR 143: 641-645
41. Lawson JP (1986) Thalassemia, in radiology, diagnosis, imaging, intervension, Taveras and Ferrucci, vol. 5. Lippincott and Harper Philadelphia, pp 1-7
42. Leccisotti A, Meloni T (1967) Sui rapporti fra le alteraziono ossee e la maturazione scheletrica nell' anemia mediterranea. Nunt Radiol 33: 179-202
43. Logothetis J, Loewenson RB, Augoustaki O, Economidou J, Costantoulakis M (1972) Body growth in Cooley's anemia (homozygous beta-thalassemia) with correlative study as to other aspects of the illness in 138 cases. Pediatrics 50: 92-99
44. Logothetis J, Economidou J, Costantoulakis M, Augoustaki O, Loewenson RB, Bilek M (1971) Cephalofacial derformities in thalassemia major (Cooley's anemia). AM J Dis Child 121: 300-306
45. Long JA, Doppman JL, Nienhuis AW (1980) Computed tomographic studies of thoracic extramedullary hematopoieses, J Comput Assa Tom 4: 67-70
46. Lucarelli G,Polchi P, Galimberti M, Delfini C, Giardini C, Angelucci E, Politi P, Baronciani D, Manenti F, La Nasa G (1985) Trapianto di midollo osseo nella thalassemia, Haematologica (Pavia) 70: 407-413
47. Masera G (1985) La terapia delle talassemie. Regime transfusionale: aspetti clinici. Haematologica (Pavia) 70: 377-381
48. Miniero R, Sacchetti L, Isolato V((1977) L'accresimento staturo-ponderale nella β-talassemia omozigote in rapporto al regime transfusionale. Min Ped 29: 73-79
49. Model B, Berdoukas V (1984) The clinical approach to thalassemia. Grune and Stratton, London
50. Montuori R, de Ritis V, Lupi L, di Girolamo R, Quattrin N (1977) Lo scheletro nella microcitemia e nella microdrepanocitosi. Rilievi dello studio di 133 casi. Atti XXVII Congr Naz Soc Ital Ematol, Torino
51. Morgan DB (1973) The metacarpal bone: a comparison of the various indices for the assessment of the amount of bone and for the detection of loss of bone. Clin Radiol 24: 77-82
52. Moseley JE (1963) Bone changes in hematologic disorders, Grune and Stratton, New York
53. Moseley JE (1974) Skeletal changes in the anemias. Semin Roentgenol 9: 169-195
54. Orsini A, Perrimond H, Pierron HH, Charvet JP, Sebag F, Rebuffel P (1973) Risultati a lungo termine della terapia del morbo di Cooley. Prospect Pediatr 11: 415-421
55. Ortolani M, Cremonese M (1963) Le alterazioni scheletriche nel morbo die Cooley. Clin Ortop 15: 599-614
56. Orzincolo C, Castaldi G, Scutellari PN, Bariani L, Pinca A (1986) Aseptic necrosis of femoral head complicating thalassemia. Skeletal Radiol 15: 541-544
57. Papavasiliou CG (1965) Tumor simulating intrathoracic extramedullary hemopoiesis. Clinical and roentgenologic considerations. AJR 93: 695-702
58. Papavasiliou C, Gouliamos A, Andreou J (1986) The marrow heterotopia in thalassemia. Eur J Radiol 6: 92-96
59. Papavasiliou C, Konstantoulakis M, Priovolos J, Labrakos E, Agrogiannis B, Manettas E, Papaodysseas S, Pippis P (1979) The anterior costal margin mass in patients with thalassemia major. Clin Radiol 30: 521-524
60. Piomelli S, Danoff SJ, Becker MH, Lipera MJ, Travis SF (1969) Prevention of bone malformations and cardiomegaly in Cooley's anemia by early hypertransfusion regimen, Ann NY Acad Sci 165: 427-436
61. Piomelli S, Karpatkin MH, Arzanian M, Zamani M, Becker MH, Geneiser N, Danoff SJ, Kuhns WJ (1974) Hypertransfusion regimen in patients with Cooley's anemia. Ann NY Acad Sci 232: 186-192

62. Resnick D (1981) Hemoglobinopathies and other anemias. In: Resnick D, Niwayama G (eds.) Diagnosis of bone and joint disorders. Saunders, Philadelphia
63. Rodolico G, Cavallaro V, Minutolo V, Di Cataldo A (1985) La splenectomia nel trattamento della talassemia. Haematologica (Pavia) 70: 399–405
64. Russo G (1985) Terapia ferrochelante della talassemia. Haematologica (Pavia) 70: 391-398
65. Schorr JB, Radel E (1964) Transfusion therapy and its complications in patients with Cooley's anemia. Ann NY Acad Sci 119: 703–708
66. Scutellari PN, Bighi S, Franceschini F, Orzincolo C (1982) Le alterazioni scheletriche delle betatalassemie intermedie, Studio clinico e radiologico. Minn Med 73: 457–466
67. Scutellari PN, Bighi S, Orzincolo C, Nibbio A (1981) Stato attuale delle alterazioni scheletriche delle beta-talassemie. Riv Emoter Immunoematol 28: 39–66
68. Scutellari PN, Franceschini F, Orzincolo C (1981) Skeletal changes in treated β-thalassemias: a reappraisal. Rays 7: 13–25
69. Scutellari PN, Orzincolo C, Bighi S (1981) Studio xeroradiografico delle alterazioni ossee nelle beta-talassemie. Radiol Med (Torino) 67: 913-919
70. Scutellari PN, Orzincolo C, Calzolari F (1983) Aspetti radiologici delle alterazioni odonto-stomatologiche nellβ-talassemie. Minerva Stomatol 32: 433–440
71. Scutellari PN, Orzincolo C, Calzolari F, Tilotta F (1983) Le coste nelle β-talassemie. Evoluzione delle alterazioni in rapporto alla terapia transfusionale. Radiol Med (Torino) 69: 654–660
72. Scutellari PN, Orzincolo C, Tamarozzi R (1985) Xeradiography in β-thalassemia. Skeletal Radiol 13: 39–43
73. Silvestroni E, Bianco I, Brancati C (1971) Le emoglobinopatie mediterranee. Recenti Progr Med 51: 212–249
74. Tas I, Smith P, Cohen T (1976) Metric and morphologic characteristic of the dentition in beta thalassaemia major in man. Arch Oral Biol 21: 583–586
75. Toti A (1951) Le fratture traumatiche del morbo die Cooley. Ann Radiol (Bologna) 23: 81–92
76. Vullo C (1981) Treatment and prognosis of thalassemias, Haematologica 66: 293–308
77. Weatherall DJ, Clegg JB (1981) the thalassaemia syndromes.Blackwell Scientific Oxford
78. Weatherall DJ, Clegg JB (1982) Thalassaemia revisited. Cell 29: 7–9
79. Wolff JA, Luke KH (1969) Management of thalassaemia. A comparative programm. Ann NY Acad Sci 165: 423–426
80. Wolman IJ (1964) Transfusion therapy in Cooley's anemia: growth and health as related to long-range hemoglobin levels. A progress report. Ann NY Acad Sci 119: 736–747
81. Solmann IJ, Ortoloani M (1969) Some clinical features of Cooley's anemia patients as related to transfusion schedules. Ann NY Acad Sci 165: 407–414
82. Zaino EC (1980) Pathophysiology of thalassemia. Ann NY Acad Sci 344: 284–303
83. Zaino EC, Kuo B, Roginsky MS (1969) Growth retardation in thalassemia major. Ann NY Acad Sci 165: 394–399

7 Grading System of Osseous Changes in Thalassemia

E. H. Hassanein and M. I. Gharib

The radiological changes encountered in thalassemia and its variants involve many organs. There is general agreement to group these changes into two main categories: osseous and extraosseous manifestations.

The underlying pathogenesis of both osseous and extraosseous radiological findings is mainly the state of chronic hemolytic anemia that exists in different degrees of severity according to the type of thalassemia. This state of chronic hemolytic anemia will lead to compensatory bone marrow hyperplasia, together with extramedullary hemopoiesis, on the one hand, and to certain complications caused by the anemia, hemosiderin deposition and small vascular occlusions on the other.

Since the first detailed description of radiological bone change in thalassemia by Cooley et al. in 1925 and 1927 [1, 2], a number of reports and publications have followed, covering these changes from various aspects, as well as in relation to certain parameters [3–13].

The main and most manifest osseous changes, in the form of decreased bone density and wide bone marrow spaces and medullary cavities, are due to bone marrow hyperplasia as a compensatory mechanism to the existing chronic hemolytic anemia. Another finding – the occurrence of pathological fractures, including asymptomatic compression fractures of the vertebral bodies – can also be related to bone marrow hyperplasia. Premature epiphyseal fusion of the long bones has been described, but its cause and pathogenesis have not been well defined.

Grading of Individual Bone Changes

A skeletal survey is always required to recognise the osseous changes in thalassemia patients. Such a survey should cover four parts: (a) skull and facial bones; (b) small tubular bones of the hands and feet; (c) long bones; and (d) axial skeleton – the spine, ribs, scapulae and pelvis.

In a attempt to grade osseous changes in the skull in thalassemia, Gawad et al. [14] considered two measurements: (a) maximum thickness of the skull vault in the frontal region on the standard lateral skull radiogram, and (b) interorbital distance between the most convex points along the medial margins of the orbital bony cavities on the standard occipitofrontal skull radiogram.

In a clinical study on 39 patients with thalassemia (33 with thalassemia major and 6 with thalassemia intermedia) [15–17], grading of the osseous changes in each of the four parts of the skeletal survey was attempted. Four grades of severity were defined:

0: No bone changes
+: Mild bone changes
++: Moderate bone changes
+++: Severe bone changes.

A summary of the severe grade (+++) of bone changes in each part is as follows:

1. *Skull, and facial bones* (Fig. 1)
- Marked cranial vault thickening, with hair-on-end pattern
- Granular rarefaction
- Overgrowth of facial bones, with obliteration of paranasal sinuses, widening of

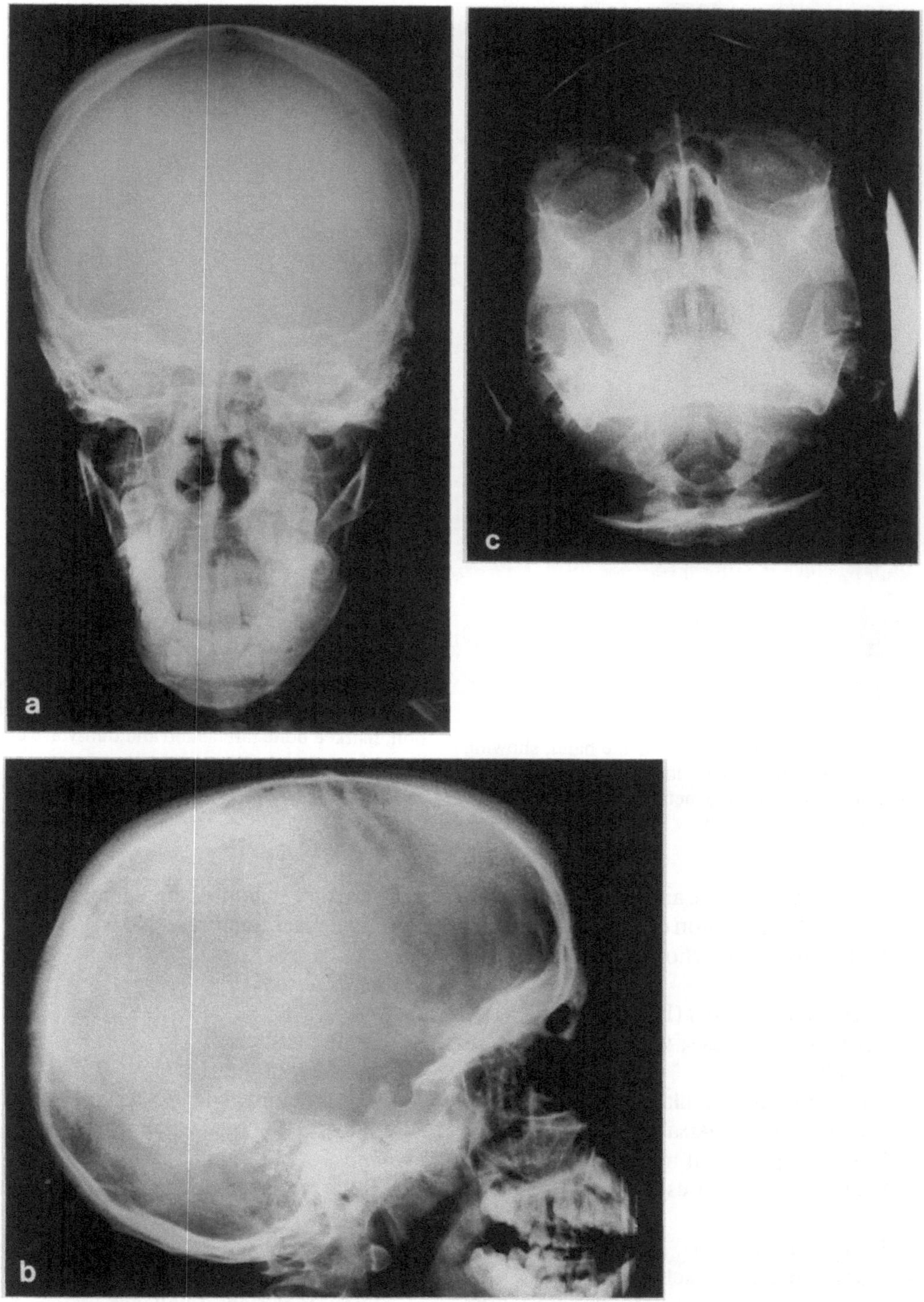

Fig. 1. a Occipitofrontal view of skull, showing bone changes in the vault. The interorbital distance is measured in this view. **b** Lateral view of skull, showing hair-on-end pattern. The maximum thickness of the frontal skull vault region is measured in this view. **c** Occipitomental view of skull, showing bony overgrowth with obliteration of the maxillary paranasal sinuses

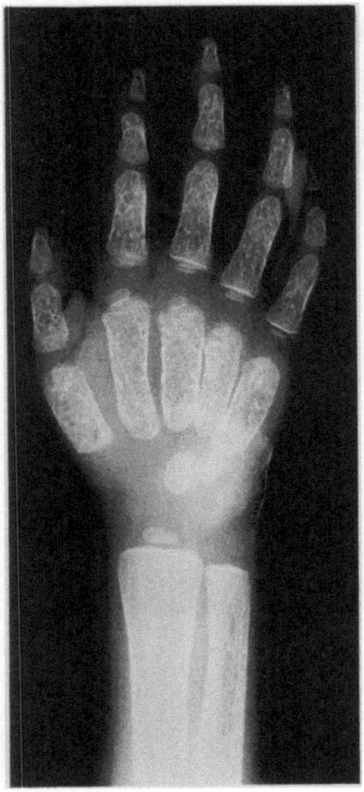

Fig. 2. Anteroposterior view of the hand, showing grade +++ bone changes in the form of expanded medullary cavities of the metacarpals and phalanges, with severe osteoporosis

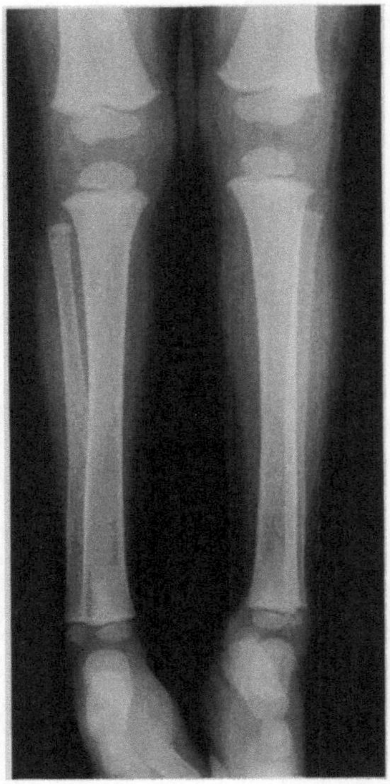

Fig. 3. Anteroposterior view of both legs, showing grade +++ bone changes, with medullary expansion, marked bone rarefaction and transverse dense lines of arrested growth

interorbital distance and overbite on lower jaw due to protrusion of the upper maxilla
- Mandibular rarefaction

2. *Small tubular bones* (Fig. 2)
- Severe osteoporosis, with coarse trabecular pattern
- Expansion of medullary cavities of metacarpals and metatarsals
- Delay in epiphyseal maturation
- Pathological fractures

3. *Long bones* (Fig. 3)
- Marked bone rarefaction
- Medullary expansion, with modelling deformities
- Trabecular bone destruction and atrophy
- Multiple transverse dense lines of arrested growth
- Premature fusion of the epiphyses
- Pathological fractures

4. *Axial skeleton* (Fig. 4)

a) *Ribs*
  - Bone rarefaction
  - Swelling of the ribs
  - Rib notching, with posterior rib expansion

b) *Spine*
  - Bone rarefaction, with coarse trabecular pattern
  - Increase in the longitudinal dimension of the vertebrae
  - Possible vertebral collapse

c) *Pelvis, and scapulae*
  - Bone rarefaction
  - Coarse bone trabeculae with characteristic fan-like striations

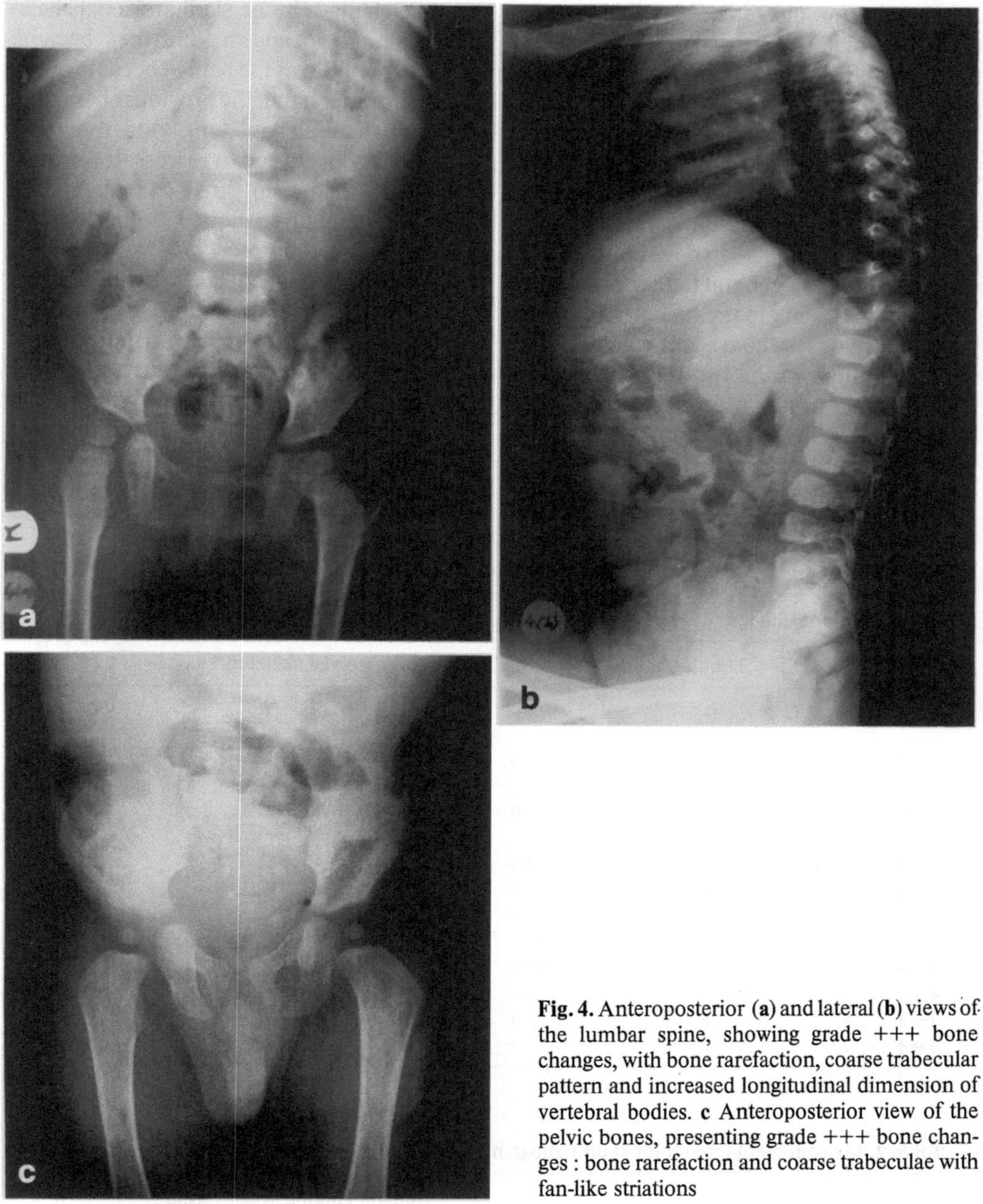

Fig. 4. Anteroposterior (**a**) and lateral (**b**) views of the lumbar spine, showing grade +++ bone changes, with bone rarefaction, coarse trabecular pattern and increased longitudinal dimension of vertebral bodies. **c** Anteroposterior view of the pelvic bones, presenting grade +++ bone changes : bone rarefaction and coarse trabeculae with fan-like striations

General Grading System

Following the grading of individual bone changes in the four parts of the skeletal survey, a general grading system was adopted. This system utilises grading of the four parts to produce a certain scale for general grading (0, +, ++, +++). The basic structure of this system is presented in Table 1. The two skull measurements - maximum frontal region thickness and interorbital distance - were correlated to the general grading system scale. The correlation proved to be valid and is presented in Table 2.

In analysing the general grading system, three main factors appeared to be responsible for the grade of severity of the osseous changes:

1. There was a definite relation between the **age of the patient** and both the severity and the pattern of bone involvement. The relation between age and the general grading scale in 12 patients is shown in Table 3, where there is a general tendency towards higher grades in older patients [15]. A certain more or less consistent pattern could be identiffied in the osseous changes. In the 1st year of life, osseous changes were usually seen in the small tubular bones of the hands and feet and in the lower thirds of both femora. With the progress of age, bone changes in the skull and axial skeleton started to appear, and they became more manifest as the patient became older. On the other hand, the previous changes in the small tubular and long bones remained stationary or started to regress. It was possible to follow up three patients and to demonstrate this pattern with the progress of age (Table 4).
This pattern may explain why the phalangeal and calvarial findings reported by Lawson et al. [18] were at variance in six of their patients. Comparing the size of the nutrient phalangeal foramina with the calvarial vascular markings, they found that three patients showed abnormal calvarial markings with normal nutrient foramina,

Table 1. Basic structure of general grading system

Degree of bone changes in each part of skeleton				General grade
Skull	Tubular bones	Long bones	Axial skeleton	
0	0	0	0	0
0	+	+	0	
+	+	+	+	+
+	0	0	0	
+	++	++	+	
++	++	++	++	++
++	+	+	+	
+++	+++	+++	+++	
+++	++	++	+++	+++
+++	+	+	++	
+++	+	+	+	

Table 2. Measurement criteria for skull radiograms correlated to general grading system scale

Measurement criterion	Normal value	General grading system scale		
		+	++	+++
Maximum thickness of frontal region on standard lateral skull radiogram	Up to 7 mm	Below 10 mm	Between 10 and 15 mm	Above 15 mm
Interorbital distance on standard occipitofrontal skull radiogram	Up to 21 mm	Below 25 mm	Between 25 and 28 mm	Aboce 28 mm

and that the situation was reversed in the other three patients. Lawson et al. correlated such variance to the age of onset of the transfusion regimen. It is, however, logical to assume that transfusion therapy increased in frequency with the advance of age. The age of the patient expresses two parameters – the duration of the disease and the onset and duration of transfusion therapy. The reported variance can thus be attributed to the changing pattern of osseous findings with advancing age described above. This pattern can be explained by the alteration of active red bone marrow in the small tubular and long bones to fatty marrow with progress of age, and the subsequent nonsharing of such fatty marrow in the compensatory hyperplasia.

2. **Form of Thalassemia** is also a factor. The incidence of bone changes among patients with thalassemia major is higher than in those with thalassemia intermedia; the degree of severity of these changes is also more marked. When severe (grade +++) bone changes exist in patients with thalassemia intermedia, an additional factor, such as the level of fetal hemoglobin (HbF) in the blood, is usually responsible.

It is thus clear that it is the degree of ineffective erythropoiesis that determines

Table 3. Correlation between patient's age and general grading scale in 12 representative cases

Form of thalassemia	Patient no.	General grading scale	Patient's age
	1	0	4.5 months
	2	0	6.0 months
	3	+	1.5 years
	4	+	1.5 years
Thalassemia major	5	++	3.0 years
	6	++	3.0 years
	7	+++	4.0 years
	8	+++	5.0 years
Thalassemia intermedia	1	0	18.0 years
	2	+	11.0 years
	3	+	6.0 years
	4	+++	17.0 years

Table 4. Pattern of osseous with progress of age in three patients

Patient no.	Age at examination and follow-up(s)	Radiological changes			
		Skull	Small tubular	Long bones	Axial skeleton
1	1.0 year	0	+	+	0
	3.0 years	+	+	+	+
	3.5 years	++	+	+	++
2	1.5 years	++	++	++	+
	3.0 years	+++	+	+	++
3	2.0 years	+	+	+	+
	4.0 years	++	+	+	+

Table 5. Severity of osseous changes in 13 patients with HbF levels ranging from 90% to 100%

Age group	No. of cases	Mean Hb in 100 ml	No. of cases in general grading scale			
			0	+	++	+++
Below 1 year	4	5.8	2	2	0	0
1–2 year	2	3.8	0	0	2	0
Above 2 years	7	4.9	0	0	0	7[a]

[a] One of these patients was a 17-year-old male with thalassemia intermedia.

the severity of bone changes, rather than the type or stage of chronic hemolytic anemia.

3. There is a definite correlation between the **increased level of HbF** in the blood and the general grading scale of osseous changes, provided that the age of the patient is above 1 year.
The relationship between the grading system and age is shown in Table 5 for 13 patients with HbF level ranging between 90% and 100%. All were thalassemia major patients except for a 17-year-old male with thalassemia intermedia. It is noteworthy that HbF viewed as a percentage of total Hb is an insufficient indicator of severity when taken alone. It is more accurate to consider the level of total Hb and the percentage of HbF. This is clear in Table 5, where total Hb ranges between 3,8 and 5,8 g/100 ml, with HbF ranging between 90% and 100% of this low total value. All seven patients above 2 years old, including the thalassemia intermedia patient, presented grade +++ bone changes. The two patients aged 1 and 2 years showed grade ++ osseous changes, and this was expected in this age group. The remaining four patients were all below 1 year of age. Two showed grade + tubular and long bone changes, while the other two were grade 0 with no osseous changes.
This relationship can explain why in most patients with thalassemia intermedia, osseous changes of only grade + could be noted, as the mean HbF level is usually around 20%. The only patient with thalassemia intermedia who presented grade +++bone changes had a HbF level of 90%.
The relationship between the HbF level and the grading scale of osseous changes in thalassemia can be explained by the pathophysiological aspect of thalassemia described by Weatherall [19]. He stated that HbF has a high oxygen affinity; in the presence of anemia in these patients, this will result in tissue hypoxia, which is the main factor in stimulating erythropoietin production. This will lead to bone marrow hyperplasia and subsequent osseous changes.

It would be fair to assume that the osseous changes in thalassemia can be correlated to a number of parameters that are inidicative of the type and progress of the disease. A grading system for these changes is obviously related to the three main categories of thalassemia: minor, intermedia and major. However, it is the degree of inefficient erythropoiesis that is actually related to the grading scale. The general grading scale can translate fairly well the duration of the disease, which expresses two parameters: the age of the patient and the frequency of the infusion therapy regimen. The level of HbF in the blood is an evident underlying factor in the severity of osseous changes in patients above 1 year of age. The level of HbF should be considered both absolutely, in grams per 100 millilitres and as a percentage of the total Hb value, which is usually low in patients with chronic haemolytic anemia.

References

1. Cooley TD,Lee P (1925) A series of cases of splenomegaly in children with anemia and peculiar bone changes. Transactions of the American Pediatric Society, 37: 29–38
2. Cooley TD, Witwer ER, Lee P (1927) Anemia in children with splenomegaly and peculiar changes in bones: report of cases. Am J Dis Child 34: 347–363
3. Caffey J (1951) Cooley's erythroblastic anemia, some skeletal findings in adolescents and young adults. A J R Radiat Ther 65: 547–560
4. Caffey J (1957) Cooley's anemia: a review of the roentgenographic findings in the skeleton. Am J R Radiat Ther 78: 381–391
5. Baker DH (1964) Roentgen manifestations of Cooley's anemia. Ann N Y Acad Sci 119: 641–661
6. Carrarino G, Erlandosn E (1964) Premature fusion of epiphysis in Cooley's anemia. Radiology 83: 565–664
7. Middlemiss JM, Raper AB (1966) Skeletal changes in the haemoglobinopathies. J Bone Joint Surg (Br) 48: 693–702
8. Bohrer SP (1970) Acute long bone diaphyseal infarcts in sickle cell disease. Br J Radiol 43: 685–697
9. Poznanski AK (1974) The hand and radiologic diagnosis. Saunders, Philadelphia, PP 489–491
10. Dines DM, Canale VC, Arnalde WD (1976) Fractures in thalassemia. J Bone Joint Sur 58: 662–666
11. Cockshott WP, Middlemiss H (1979) Clinical radiology in the tropics. Churchill-Livingston, New York, p 77
12. Lawson JP, Abcow RC, Pearson HA (1981) The ribs in thalassemia. 1. The relationship to therapy. Radiology 140: 663–672
13. Fink IJ, Pastakia B, Barranger JA (1984) Enlarged phalangeal nutrient foramina in Gaucher disease and β-thalassemia major. A J R 143: 647–649
14. Gawad MA, Safouh MA, Aeda M et al. (1975) Thalassemia in Qatar. Egypt J Radiol Nucl Med 6: 109–119
15. Gharib MI (1978) Radiological survey of bone marrow changes in thalassemia. Thesis in Radiodiagnosis, Faculty of Medicine, University of Alexandria, Alexandria
16. Elsheikh SO, Gharib MI, Zaky H, Hassanein EH (1981) Osseous changes in thalassemia. Egypt J Radiol Nucl Med 12: 23–31
17. Gharib MI, Hassanein EH (1986) A proposed grading of radiographic changes in thalassemia. Proc 32nd natl congr, Mediterranean meetings of radiology, Italian association of radiology and nuclear medicine, Milan, June 1986
18. Lawson JP, Albow RC, Pearson MA (1984) Clavarial and phalangeal vascular impressions in thalassemia. A J R 143: 641–645
19. Weatherall DJ (1976) The thalssemia: genetic and pathophysiological aspects. Postgrad Med J (Suppl) 2: 52–63

8 Computed Tomography Evaluation of the Upper Abdomen in β-Thalassemia

A. D. Gouliamos

Introduction

Clinical management of β-thalassemia depends on repeated blood transfusions and on chelation therapy. Computed tomography (CT) can provide the opportunity to relate CT density to iron deposition; therefore, CT appearance may be essential for evaluation of abdominal organs for the degree of hemochromatosis.

Subsequent to chronic transfusion therapy, red blood cells are lysed, and iron is deposited in the liver and spleen. When iron load is excessive, iron may be found in parenchymal cells as well. Drainage to adjacent lymph nodes will occasionally follow. Iron deposition in the tissues explains the high attenuation value seen in the liver, spleen, and lymph nodes in these patients.

Not only density changes, but also volume changes in abdominal organs and lymph nodes can be studied by CT in patients with β-thalassemia. Specific changes have been described in the liver, spleen, pancreas, adrenals, bowel, kidneys and abdominal lymph nodes [1, 2, 5].

The reason for increased iron deposition may be related to the transfusion treatment program. The enormous body load of iron, which accumulates in this condition, is stored largely in the reticuloendothelial tissues. Iron accumulates as a result of hemolysis and increased iron absorption from the bowel and from blood transfusions. It has been estimated that most patients with thalessemia receive 4–8 g iron per year from blood transfusion and excrete 3–4 g of this with the help of a chelating agent, desferrioxamine. The remaining iron is deposited in the reticuloendothelial system. Excess iron is deposited in a protein-bound form as ferritin and hemosiderin. It is evident that the duration of anemia is critical in the evolution of radiological findings.

The unique feature of the CT scanner is that it presents an absolute value of the attenuation coefficient (μ) for each element. The attenuation properties of a material depend on two parameters, density and atomic (chemical) composition. As the atomic number increases, so does the attenuation, particularly for higher elements such as iron, where photoelectric absorption becomes dominant.

The quantitative information contained in a CT image has been used for a variety of studies, including bone and soft tissue densitometry, organ sizing, and contrast enhancement measurement. Of course, it is important to know that many factors influence CT values, including scan noise, tissue noise, variation of machine performance, movement, and contrast artifacts.

In the computed tomogram, increased iron content (and cirrhosis) causes a distinct increase in the density of abdominal organs. A detailed description of the findings in each of the above organs follows.

Liver

Plain X-ray films of the abdomen show enlargement of the liver, while CT evaluation demonstrates high density. μ values for normal liver parenchyma of an adult can vary between 40 and 80 HU.This value is increased in cases of iron deposition (Fig.1): at 100–140 HU, it is frequently twice the nor-

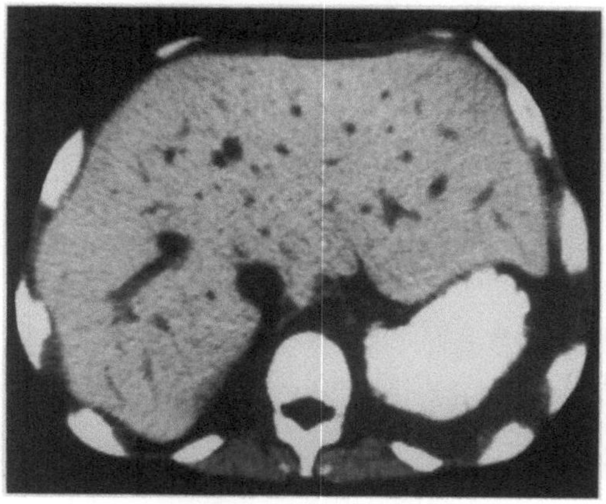

Fig. 1. Increased density due to hemochromatosis within the entire liver parenchyma (90 HU). The liver is enlarged and splenectomy has been performed

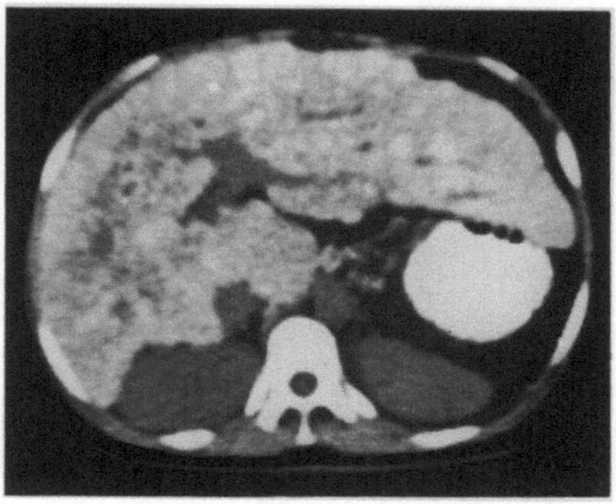

Fig. 2. Nonhomogeneous increased density within the liver parenchyma (101 HU), consistent with hemochromatosis and fibrosis

mal density value. In these cases, the liver cell contains 1–10 mg iron per 100 g tissue, i.e., 5–50 times the normal values. Hemosiderin is responsible for cellular damage and subsequent fibrosis (Fig. 2). This situation may finally evolve into cirrhotic reorganization (Fig. 3), which can be recognized by CT scan.

Liver iron content can be estimated and measured by percutaneous biopsy with a Menghini needle. CT values represent a satisfactory alternative and a noninvasive method of assessing liver iron [3]. A needle biopsy usually samples a single random area in the periphery of the right lobe of the liver, while CT measurements are representative of the entire liver parenchyma. The mean CT values from several liver scans are a good predictor of iron content. Individual sample values are less reliable. It is important to obtain a mean value from as large a number of scans as possible. This is important because values in different areas of the same organ vary widely. Dual-energy CT scanning has also been advocated for noninvasive quantification of liver iron [9]. Without exposing patients to ionizing radiation, magnetic resonance imaging (MRI) offers the potential for detection, localization, and rough quantification of the biochemical changes associated with hemosiderosis [10]. An example of liver changes in MRI is presented in Fig. 4.

Hepatic abscesses may also occur in patients with hemochromatosis. Abscess cavities usually contain pus and cellular debris; gas is present in a minority of cases. The margins of an abscess may be smooth or shaggy. An inflammatory reaction is often present in the surrounding parenchyma. CT appearance of an abscess varies according to morphological characteristics and composition. The density can be close to that of water or in the same range as those of solid tumors. Among the types of lesions that occasionally resemble hepatic abscesses are simple and parasitic cysts, hematomas, and cavitary neoplasms. In most cases, differential diagnosis between inflammatory and neoplastic lesions can be made on the basis of the clinical picture. The important aspect of CT-guided diagnostic aspiration and drainage has also been well established.

Spleen

The spleen may be involved in a large number of systemic disorders, most of which cause diffuse microscopic changes that may be either undetectable by CT or reflected in changes in size or attenuation values. Among

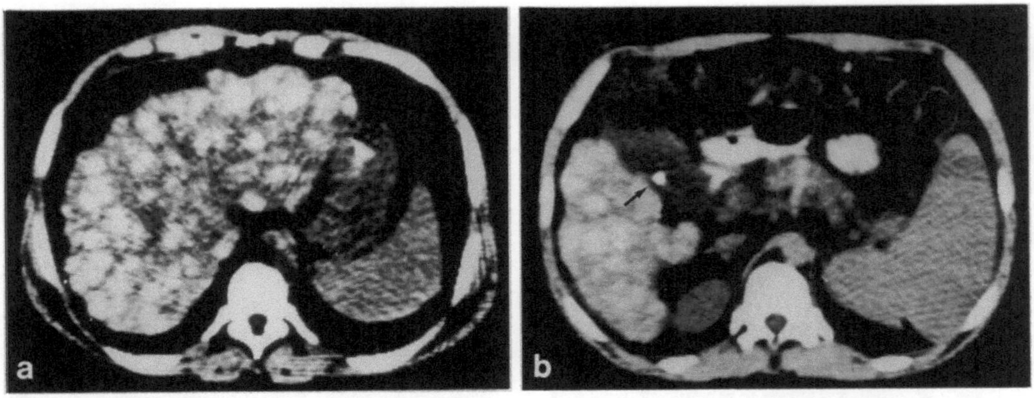

Fig. 3 a, b. Hyperdense nodules within the liver parenchyma, in adjacent sections, secondary to cirrhosis. In **b**, gall bladder calculi are also noted (*arrow*)

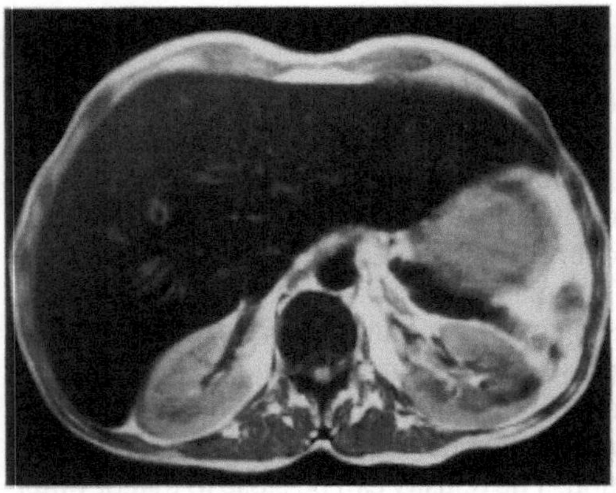

Fig. 4. MR image shows diffuse decreased signal intensity in the liver, corresponding to the presence of intracellular iron ("black" liver)

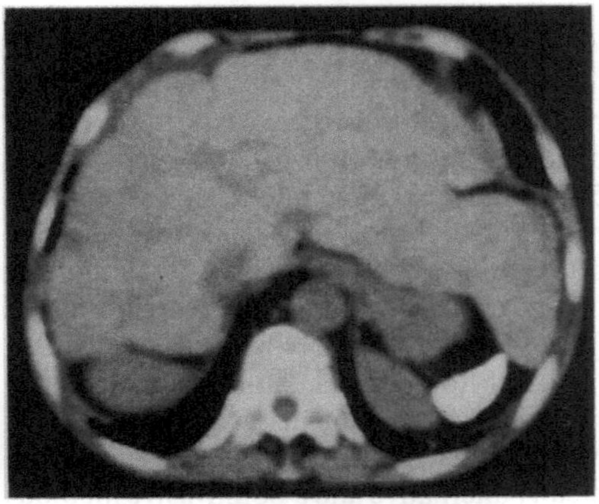

Fig. 5. Small, densely calcified spleen

the hematological diseases that may involve the spleen are thalassemia, sickle cell anemia, autoimmune hemolytic anemia, polycythemia vera, thrombocytopenic purpura, hypersplenism, and agnogenic myeloid metaplasia. In the majority of these disorders, the spleen is enlarged, its size depending on the severity and chronicity of the disease. In chronic forms of some hematological diseases and those associated with the status of intrasplenic vascular channels, the spleen may decrease in size secondary to diffuse infarction.

On histological examination splenic tissue reveals heavy iron deposition predominantly in the red pulp, with sparing of the white pulp. The iron is concentrated in prominent sinusoidal lining cells, imparting a ringlike configuration to cross-sectional views of sinusoids.

Noncontrast CT scans through the upper abdomen show splenic enlargement and increased density; the latter involves diffusely the entire spleen. Areas of decreased density can be also seen within the spleen due to erythropoietic foci.

Sickle cell anemia is known to produce small, densely calcified spleens (Fig. 5), correlating with the sequence of early infarction and fibrosis that produces functional autosplenectomy [4]. These patients are also

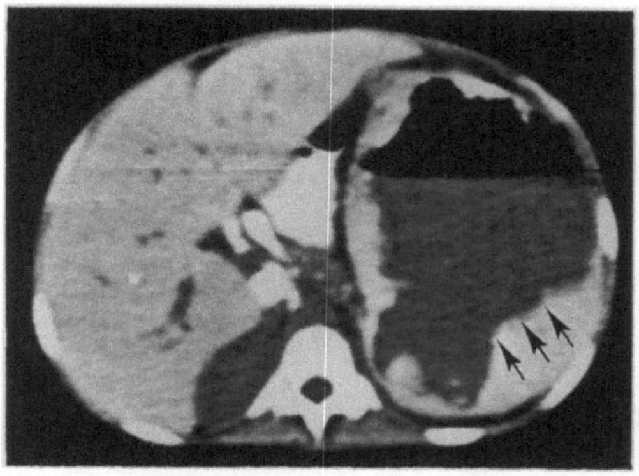

Fig. 6. Splenic abscess (*arrows*), associated with diffuse increased density in the liver parenchyma (91 HU)

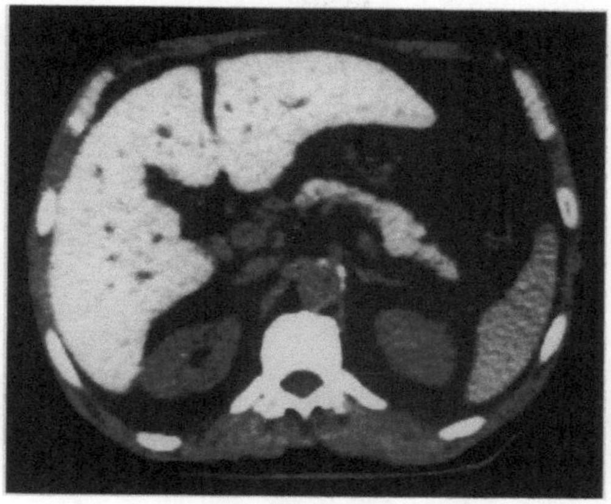

Fig. 7. Increased density in the liver and the pancreas consistent with hemochromatosis

prone to infection, which may lead to splenic abscess (Fig. 6). The presence of gas within a fluid collection is the only CT finding specific for an abscess. An intrasplenic abscess may occasionally be detected by CT but may not be visible or palpable on surgical inspection. Similar findings may be seen in patients with thalassemia, but this has not yet been reported.

Nonspecific enlargement of the spleen with perservation of its normal homogeneity may also be seen in portal venous hypertension and in splenic venous occlusion. Massive splenomegaly may also be found in the lipoidoses, including Gaucher's disease and Niemann-Pick disease. In most cases of nonspecific splenomegaly, the cause is suggested by clinical factors or by associated findings on CT or other imaging procedures. CT is capable of accurately estimating volume and is therefore helpful in the follow-up of these patients because progression or regression of splenomegaly may reflect the course of the disease and the success of therapy.

Pancreas

An increase in density of the pancreas, due to iron accumulation (Fig. 7), has been observed in a number of patients with β-thalassemia. The density of the pancreas did not exceed that of the liver. Increased density of the pancreas does not appear to correlate with pancreatic insufficiency or fibrosis.

Ultrasonography has also been used for the assessment of iron load in the pancreas. After many years of transfusion, a normal-sized but highly echogenic pancreas has been found [11].

Gall Bladder

Although there are other imaging modalities more effective and less costly than CT for visualization of the gall bladder, cholelithiasis can be demonstrated during a survey of the upper abdomen (Fig. 8). Usually, multiple radiopaque stones are demonstrated within the gall bladder or in the bile ducts when the bladder has been removed.

Adrenals

In a quarter of patients with thalassemia major, increased density of the adrenal glands can be noted. There is no direct relation between the density and the presence of adrenal insufficiency [6].

Nonneoplastic masses of the adrenal glands may occasionally appear with increased density and should be considered in the differential diagnosis. The most com-

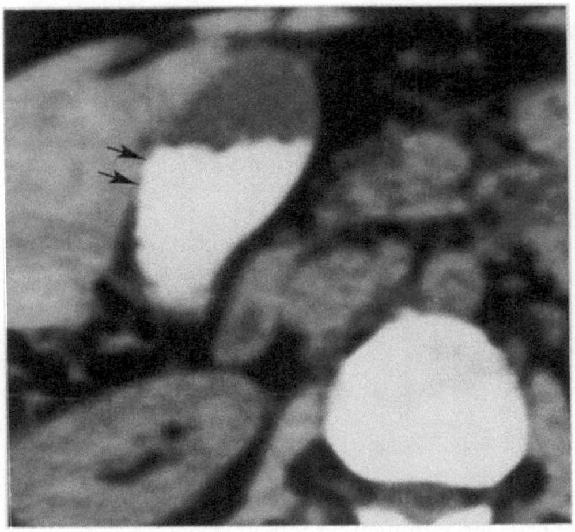

Fig. 8. Increased density in the lower portion of the gall bladder due to cholelithiasis (*arrows*)

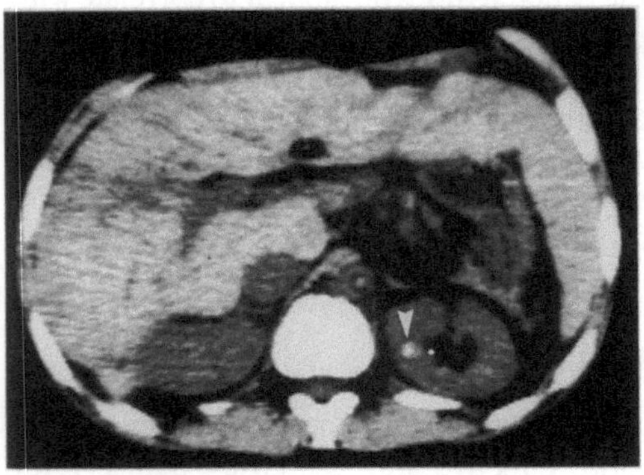

Fig. 9. Calcification in the left kidney (*arrowhead*) with associated hepatomegaly

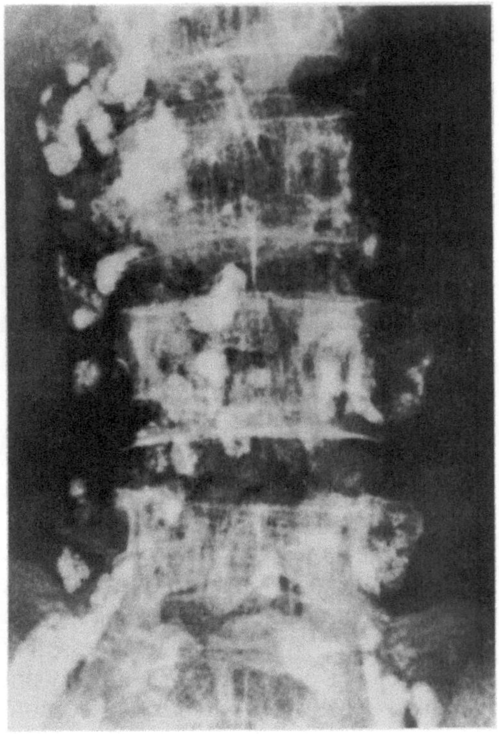

Fig. 10. Lymphogram of adult thalassemic patient, showing multiple filling defects throughout the abdominal nodes. Characteristic bone changes of the disease are present. (Reproduced with permission from Clinical Radiology [14])

mon has been adrenal gland myelolipoma, hemorrhage or hematoma, which is sometimes associated with calcification of all or portions of the gland. The calcification can be discovered originally on plain X-ray films of the abdomen.

Gastrointestinal Tract

In a small percentage of patients, there is evidence of increased density of the stomach wall and duodenum. Naturally, this finding is observed in upper abdominal scans without previous administration of contrast material. The increased density is diffuse and evenly distributed. Increased density may also be observed in the ileum.

Kidney

Large renal outlines have been observed on abdominal films of patients with thalassemia major, without evidence of urinary tract complaints [12]. Enlargement of the kidneys has been attributed to tubular dilatation; it is symmetrical, and the normal renal shape is maintained.

Deposition of iron in the kidneys is a regular feature, although the amount deposited is relatively small as compared with that in other parenchymatous organs. Extramedullary blood formation, fibrosis, and scarring may occur but are considered insignificant. Minimal focal hemosiderosis may occasionally produce elevation of CT values within the renal parenchyma (Fig. 9).

Besides thalassemia, early stages of sickle cell disease may produce large kidneys.

Lymph Nodes

Surgeons attempting therapeutic splenectomy in thalassemia major are familiar with enlarged purple abdominal lymph nodes. On section, these nodes have been shown to contain hemosiderin and erythropoietic foci [5, 13].

Increased density of lymph nodes has been noted on plain X-ray films of the abdomen in thalassemia major. This proved to be due to iron deposition. Plain X-ray films of the abdomen are usually obtained in this group of patients to detect gallstones and to study the thoracolumbar spine for fracture. In patients with thalassemia, elongated nodular densities are visualized in a chainlike fashion bilaterally along the upper lumbar and lower thoracic spine. In the lateral projection, the soft tissue radiopacities are just anterior to the vertebrae. Osteoporosis is present in the vertebrae, presumably secondary to medullary expansion. Anterior scalloping of the vertebral bodies can be seen where the nodular densities abut upon the spine. The most severely involved lymph nodes are in the chest, in the abdomen, and along the vertebral column. They may measure 2–4 cm in their greatest dimension.

The lymphographic appearance of abdominal lymph nodes in thalassemia major has been described [14]. Nodal filling defects were noted in all patients. The extra-aortic nodes are affected more markedly than iliac nodes, but both regions may be involved to some extent. The rounded, translucent areas within the contrast-filled nodes lie both centrally and peripherally; they measure 1–5 mm in diameter. There is a gradual change from coarsely granular nodes to those with multiple measurable translucent defects. Single or multiple defects may be observed. Single defects may enlarge to such a degree that the contrast medium occupies only a peripheral crescent. Multiple defects retain their rounded outline as discrete entities which are often seen in contact with each other (Fig. 10).

Pathological data from examination of abnormal nodes suggest that 24% of their dry weight is due to iron content, while calcium content is only 0,27%. This proves that the radiodensity of the lymph nodes is caused by iron storage and not by dystrophic calcification; absorption spectrophotometry data support these findings.

Because of its sensitivity to tissue densities, CT has clearly demonstrated increased attenuation caused by iron pigment in the reticuloendothelial system. Lymph node attenuation coefficients measure 145–205 HU. Since the atomic number of calcium [20] is close to that of iron [26], the lymph nodes appear "calcified".

There are other pathological processes causing a lymphographic nodal appearance similar to that in thalassemia major. Similar nodal defects can be demonstrated in cases of metastatic malignant disease and lymphomatous conditions. Other possibilities include tuberculosis, sarcoidosis, multiple myeloma, Whipple's disease, amyloidosis and Waldenström's macroglobulinemia. Therefore, difficulties regarding differential diagnosis may arise in patients suffering simultaneously from thalassemia and some other systemic disease affecting the lymph nodes. In cases of thalassemia, follow-up films at close intervals may not show evolution, while in metastatic disease or lymphoma there will be progress of the radiological findings or regression due to therapy.

Summary

Patients with β-thalassemia can be studied using CT for the possibility of discovering hemochromatosis or extramedullary hemopoieses. Volume and density changes of abdominal organs and lymph nodes can be identified. Specific findings in the liver, spleen, pancreas, adrenals, bowel, kidneys, and abdominal lymph nodes have been described.

References

1. Long JA, Doppman JL, Nienhuis AW and Mills SR (1980) Computed tomographic analysis of beta-thalassemic syndromes with hemochromatosis: pathologic findings with clinical and laboratory correlations. J Comput Assist Tomogr 4: 159–165
2. Mill SR, Doppman JL, Nienhuis AW (1977) Computed tomography in the diagnosis of excessive iron storage of the liver, J Comput Assist Tomogr 1: 101–104
3. Houang MTW, Arozena X, Skalicka A, Huehns ER (1979) Correlation between computed tomographic values and liver iron content in thalassemia major with iron overload. Lancet 1: 1322–1323
4. Magid D, Fishman EK, Siegelman SS (1984) Computed tomography of the spleen and liver in sickle cell disease. A J R 143: 245–249
5. Mitnick JS, Bosniak MA, Megibow AJ, Karpatkin M, Feiner HD, Kutin N, VanNatta F, Piomelli S (1981) CT in beta-thalassemia: iron deposition in the liver, spleen and lymph nodes. A J R 136: 1191–1194
6. Nienhuis AW, Peterson DT, Henry W (1977) Evaluation of endocrine and cardiac function in patients with iron overload on chelation therapy. In: Zaino EC (ed) Chelation therapy in chronic iron overload. Symposia Specialists
7. Champan RWG, Williams G, Bydder G, Dick R, Sherlock S, Kreel L (1980) Computed tomography for determining liver iron content in primary hemochromatosis. Br Med J 28: 440
8. Howard JM, Ghent CN, Carey LS, Flanagan PR, Valberg LS (1983) Diagnostic efficacy of hepatic computed tomography in the detection of body iron overload. Gastroenterology 84: 209
9. Goldberg HI, Cann CE, Moss AA, Ohto M, Brito A, Federle M (1982) Noninvasive quantification of liver iron in dogs with hemochromatosis using dual-energy CT scanning. Invest Radiol 17: 375–380
10. Brasch RC, Wesbey GE, Gooding CA, Koerper MA (1984) Magnetic resonance imaging of transfusional hemosiderosis complicating thalassemia major. Radiology 150: 767–771
11. Erttman R, Hausdorf G and Landbeck G (1983) Pancreatic sonography in thalassemia major. Clin Pediatr (Philadelphia) 195: 97–99
12. Grossman H, Dische R, Winchester P, Canale V (1971) Renal enlargement in thalassemia major. Radiology 100: 645–648
13. Winchester PH, Cerwin R, Dische K, Canale V (1973) Hemosiderin laden lymph nodes. A J R 118: 222–226
14. Parsons C (1977) Abdominal lymphography in thalassemia major. Clin Radiol 18: 545–548
15. Gollan JL (1983) Diagnosis of hemochromatosis. Gastroenterology 84: 418–421

9 Scintigraphic Evaluation of Organ Dysfunction in Thalassemia

J. Malamitsi

Introduction

Conventional radiology has been extensively used in assessing abnormalities caused by β-thalassemia. In contrast, there are very few references in the international literature to scintigraphic findings in this disease. Nuclear Medicine, however, offers a cheap and widely available means of evaluating functional disorders of various organs occurring in patients with this innate defect of hemopoiesis. In this chapter, the relevant literature will be reviewed. The scintigraphic images presented originate from personal data.

Hepatosplenic Scintigraphy

Many factors may cause diffuse parenchymal disorder of the liver in a patient suffering from β-thalassemia: the most important are iron overload and viral hepatitis, leading potentially to liver cirrhosis [1, 37, 55]. In addition, chronic anoxia combined with circulatory stasis and extramedullary hemopoiesis may contribute to the compromise of hepatic function [20, 36, 53]. Due to overcatabolism of bilirubin, cholelithiasis and common duct calculi are also frequent [55].

The spleen in β-thalassemia is severely affected: hyperplasia of the reticuloendothelial cells, distention of the red pulp due to phagocytosis of red blood cells, and siderosis are the main pathologic features [24].

On hepatosplenic scintigraphy both hepatomegaly and splenomegaly are noted [1, 24] (Fig. 1). In a series consisting of 30 thalassemic patients aged 4-14 years who were studied with sulfur colloid by Agnello et al. [1], the liver appeared enlarged in all cases and markedly enlarged in 23% of them. The same authors report that in 33% of the patients studied, the distribution of radiocolloid in the liver appeared homogeneous, while in the rest uptake was nonhomogeneous, with a characteristic decrease in uptake at the hilar region, attributable to hilar fibrosis. In 10% of the nonsplenectomized patients increased uptake by the spleen was observed, while in 20% of these patients bone marrow uptake appeared increased; 55% of the children were splenectomized. These scintigraphic findings - liver enlargement with nonhomogeneous uptake and increased splenic and bone marrow uptake, along with respective changes in echo structure on ultrasonography - indicate a diffuse parenchymal disorder of the liver, occasionally preceding abnormal biochemistry.

In drawing isocontour lines to estimate homogeneity in colloid uptake, Gyftaki et al. [24] reported islands of low radioactivity in central regions of the liver, which disappeared partially or totally with time. Such abnormalities of distribution were not found in normal controls. The above authors attributed these findings to the variations in blood flow and phagocytic capacity of the liver. Splenic parenchyma has equally shown islands of increased or decreased radioactivity.

On colloid scan, the spleen of β-thalassemics appears enlarged, sometimes excessively [13]. Significant decrease of splenic size has been documented following blood transfusion [4, 40, 54]: the spleen starts decreasing in size after a blood transfusion, reaching its minimum size on the 7th-10th day posttrans-

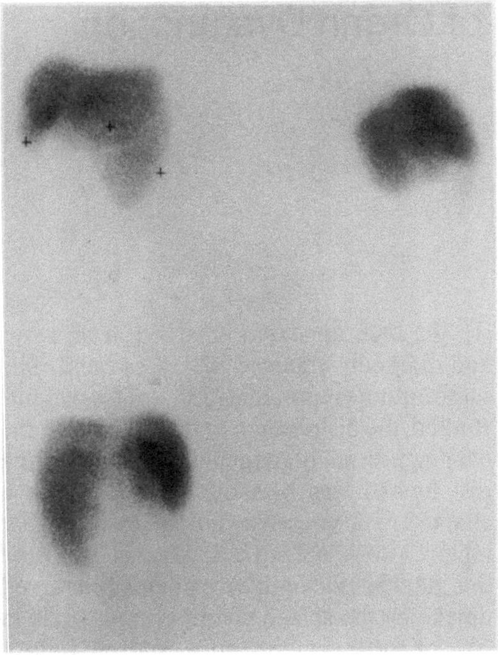

Fig. 1. Moderate hepatomegaly and excessive splenomegaly in a 23-year-old thalassemic male. Increased ^{99m}Tc-labeled phytate uptake by the spleen is noted (Anterior, right lateral and posterior views are shown).

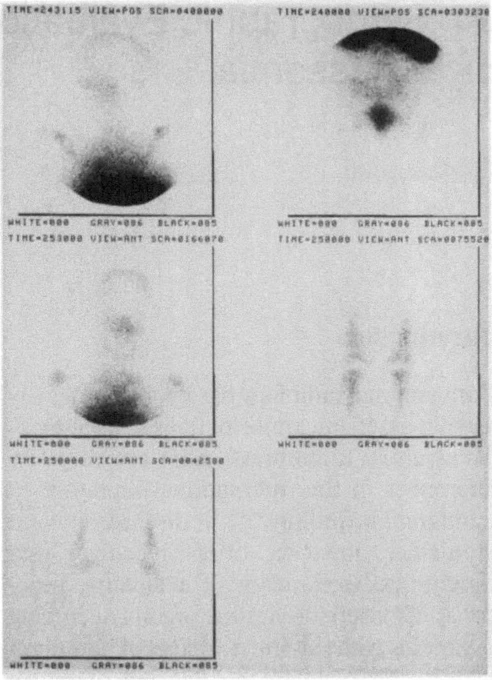

Fig. 2. Bone marrow scan using ^{99m}Tc-labeled phytate in a 22-year-old female, showing extension of marrow to the lower extremities

fusion and its maximum size before the next transfusion becomes necessary [27]. Apart from the statistically significant decrease of the scintigraphic surface of the spleen, Karpathios et al. [28] have reported significantly higher colloid uptake by the spleen in absolute terms (expressed as a percentage of total dose) 7–10 days posttransfusion. The scintigraphic changes occur mainly in the lower pole of the spleen. In the pretransfusion scan, the lower pole of the organ appears large and patchy, maximum uptake being seen in the upper pole of the organ. In the posttransfusion scan, the lower pole appears homogeneous and smaller, with a comparatively higher uptake. The authors attributed these changes to improved blood circulation in the spleen and to a greater participation of the reticuloendothelial system – in terms of number of cells – in the phagocytic function, probably due to decongestion of the splenic parenchyma after blood transfusion.

Bone Marrow Scintigraphy

In a normal adult, bone marrow – both its erythropoietic and its reticuloendothelial component – is found throughout the axial skeleton (spine, ribs, pelvis, scapula and clavicle, and variably in the skull). It extends up to the proximal part of the upper and lower extremities, i.e., the proximal one-fourth or maximally one-third of the humerus and femur [52]. In the newborn, on the contrary, hemopoietic bone marrow resides in the entire skeleton, but with advancing age it becomes limited, assuming the adult pattern around the age of 10 years [41]. Therefore, bone marrow expansion in the upper and lower extremities beyond that age is definitely abnormal.

In chronic hemolytic anemia, there is bone marrow hyperplasia [21, 22 48] and the erythropoietic and reticuloendothelial components of the marrow [52] expand to a vari-

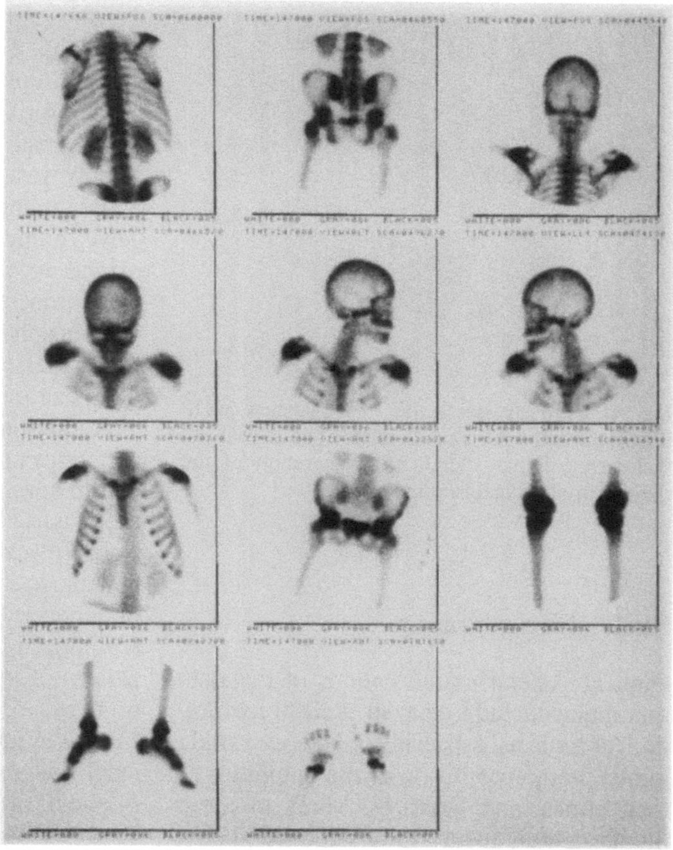

Fig. 3. Diffusely increased ^{99m}Tc-labeled methylene diphosphonate (MDP) uptake throughout the entire skeleton of a 15-year-old thalassemic male

able degree towards the periphery. In more serious cases, they extend to the small bones of the hands and feet (Fig. 2). In bone marrow scanning, either with positron-emitting ^{52}Fe for imaging of the erythropoietic component or with ^{99m}Tc-labeled colloid for imaging of the reticuloendothelial component, expansion to the extremities appears symmetrical and homogeneous. Occasionally, it may appear patchy and asymmetrical [9]. In patients with HbS β-thalassemia, bone marrow infarcts appearing as photopenic defects are frequent [7].

In chronic hemolytic anemia, bone marrow elements can also be encountered in foci of extramedullary hemopoiesis, the usual locations being in the spleen, liver, hila of kidneys, thymus gland, adrenals, pleura, appendix, retrospinal space and paraspinal region of the thorax [2, 29, 34]. Papavasiliou [43] reported ^{198}Au uptake by an extramedullary focus in the right paraspinal area in a patient with thalassemia major. A few years later, Robinson et al. [45] reported uptake of ^{59}Fe by posterior mediastinal masses of similar nature in a patient with thalassemia intermedia. On a ^{99m}Tc-labeled sulfur colloid scan, Bronn et al. [5] have shown bone marrow expansion into distal extremities and uptake in a paravertebral mass in a patient with thalassemia major, thus confirming noninvasively the radiological suspicion of extramedullary hemopoiesis. In addition, Newton et al. [39] and Sebes et al. [46] have detected pelvic sites of ectopic hemopoiesis in patients with thalassemia intermedia, using ^{99m}Tc-labeled sulfur colloid.

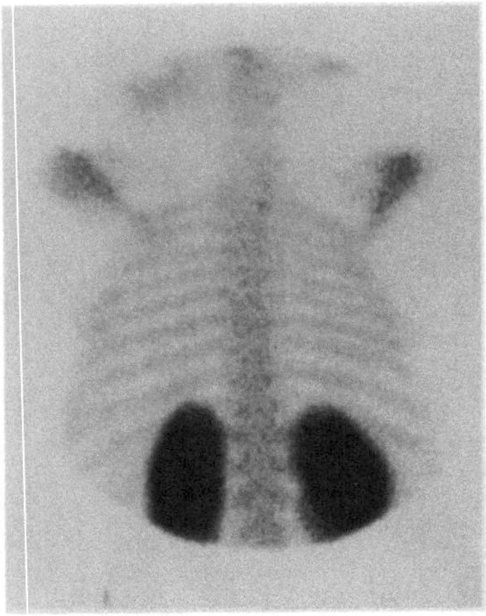

Fig. 4. Diffusely decreased ^{99m}Tc-labeled MDP uptake throughout the axial skeleton of a 21-year-old thalassemic female. High renal excretion of the radiopharmaceutical is noted

Skeletal Scintigraphy

Clinical skeletal manifestations of thalassemia major include delayed skeletal maturation; arthralgias, especially of knee and ankle joints; premature fusion of the epiphyses of long bones; and fractures. Many of these manifestations recur at the same site, being the main cause of multiple bone deformities [16].

Radiological skeletal findings in thalassemia major are those of osteopenia [3, 6]. However, histopathologic data suggest that the changes seen in many patients are of the osteomalacic type, along with iron deposition at calcium sites and findings of hyperparathyroidism [23]. According to some authors, the findings are caused by hypoparathyroidism [19, 44]. In addition, joints of thalassemic patients are affected by various types of arthritis, i.e., hemochromatosis arthritis [23, 47], gout [35, 38, 42, 49, 50], and septic arthritis [11, 26]. A particular thalassemic osteoarthropathy has also been described, appearing in the 3rd or 4th decade of life and affecting mainly the lower extremities. This osteoarthropathy may be related to the severe osteopenic or osteomalacic changes which lead to microfractures with weight bearing or minimal exercise [8].

As far as the scintigraphic appearence of the bone is concerned, increased diphosphonate uptake by the entire skeleton has been described by Zaino [55] in patients with thalassemia major. In particular, increased activity was shown in the frontal and parietal bones, mandible, sternum, ribs, vertebrae, pelvis, humerus, and femur. In contrast, Valdez and Jacobstein [51] have reported generalized decrease in uptake of ^{99m}Tc-labeled polyphosphate by the bones in four patients with thalassemia major, along with increased renal size and increased renal excretion of the radiopharmaceutical. They attributed this poor bone uptake to the marrow hyperplasia – due to severe anemia – in keeping with the radiological findings of bone marrow expansion. However, Fordham and Ali [17] believe that marrow expansion causes an appearance of increased metaphyseal uptake on bone scanning, most obvious around the knees, the pattern of uptake being that of immobilization of a patient and of osteomalacia. Increased uptake can be seen diffusely in the axial skeleton due to compression fractures of one or more vertebrae in the thoracic and lumbar regions [10]. Fractures can also be seen in the lower extremities, usually being multiple [10].

Lastly, referring to thalassemic osteoarthropathy, Gratwick observed increased radiopharmaceutical uptake on bone scintigraphy of the joints of the lower extremieties, especially the ankles; this regressed after a period of immobilization [23]. Examples of bone scintigraphy findings are seen in Figs. 2–6.

Radionuclide Ventriculography

Biventricular congestive heart failure and arrythmia are the main causes of death in thalassemic patients during adolescence or young adulthood [14, 15]. Therefore, in order to improve their prognosis, it is imperative to identify cardiac dysfunction early. Electrocardiography and chest roentgenography are

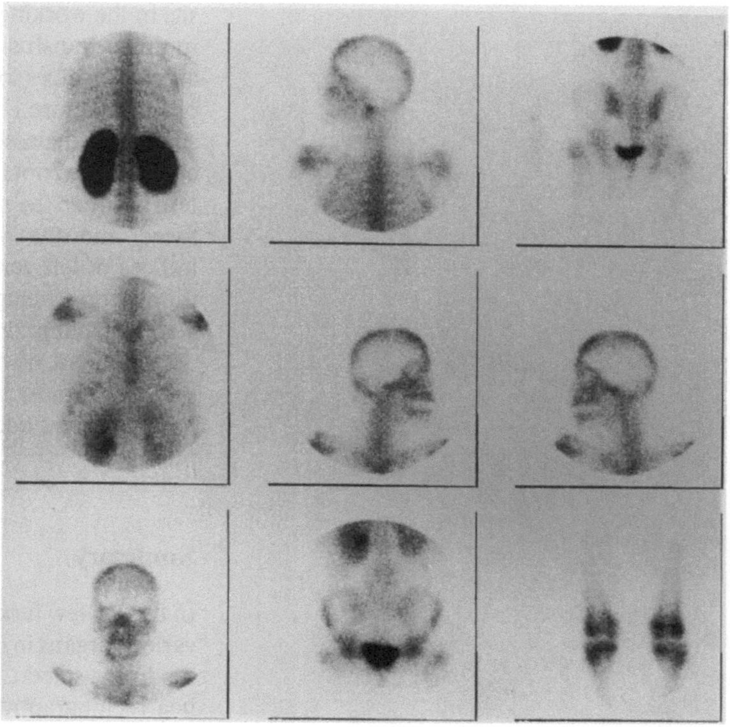

Fig. 5. Moderately diffusely decreased ^{99m}Tc-labeled MDP uptake by the skeleton, along with high excretion of the radiopharmaceutical by the enlarged kidneys in a 24-year-old thalassemic male

not very sensitive for early detection [25]. Despite the detailed anatomical and functional information offered, echocardiography performed at rest [25] and cardiac catheterization, even after application of isometric stress [12], have not proved of much help in diagnosing compromised functional reserve.

In contrast, exercise radionuclide ventriculography can reveal subclinical left ventricular failure in patients with thalassemia major, by assessing the response of the left ventricle to exercise (Fig. 7). Leon et al. [31] have shown an abnormal left ventricular ejection fraction response to exercise in thalassemic patients without a history of cardiac disease, who had a normal radionuclide ejection fraction at rest and a normal fractional shortening at rest on echocardiography. Furthermore, the same group of investigators [31] differentiated the patients according to the transfused iron load. They found that patients who had received fewer than 100 units of transfused blood had normal ejection fraction responses to exercise, whereas the majority of patients who had received more than 100 transfusions had abnormal responses. In particular, the latter group of patients had a much more pronounced average change of ejection fraction between rest and exercise than patients who had received fewer than 100 transfusions. In addition, none of the hematologic indices studied (i.e., hematocrit, serum ferritin, white cell ascorbic acid content, and urinary iron excretion) except for the total number of transfusions correlated significantly to the ejection fraction response to exercise. Lastly, in a few patients with markedly abnormal left ventricular ejection fraction during rest and exercise, regional wall motion abnormalities were detected, without evidence of significant coronary artery disease.

Freeman et al. [18] state that the majority of patients with thalassemia major – 71% of the population studied – will demonstrate abnormal left ventricular ejection fraction

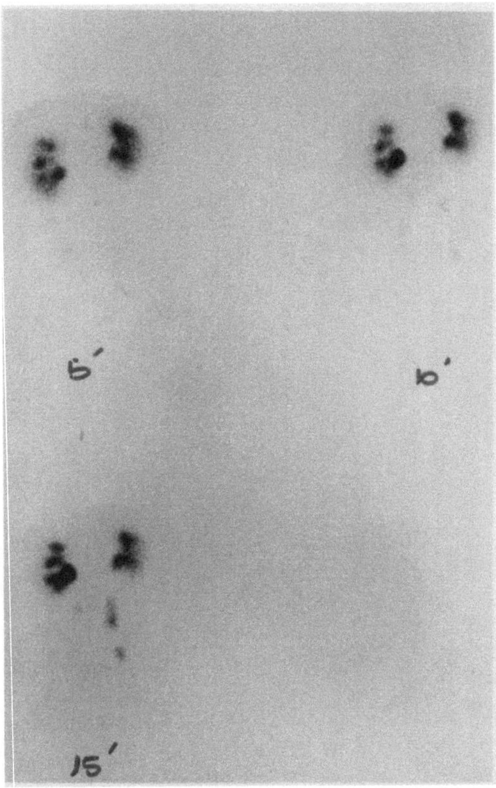

Fig. 6. Renal imaging with ^{99m}Tc-labeled MDP in the course of bone scanning in a 21-year-old thalassemic female. Enlargement of the kidneys and calyceal dilatation are seen (Images obtained at five, ten and fiften minutes postinjection)

responses to exercise, while the response is normal at rest. They also found a normal ejection fraction response in patients who had received a smaller number of transfusions (average iron load 16±2 g) and had a lower ferritin level (average values 1043±400 ng/ml). Bearing in mind that chelation therapy can lead to a negative iron balance, they went on to study a number of patients after a 1-year intensive chelation regimen with desferrioxamine. They showed that this regimen helped the patients to maintain or even improve their ventricular performance. According to Freeman et al., the above observation suggests that in early stages, i.e., before severe myocardial damage has occurred, functional abnormalities of the heart can be reversible. However, iron deposits in the working myocardium as a result of multiple transfusions are not considered by all investigators to be responsible for genesis of heart failure [15, 32, 33]. In an extensive study of 60 thalassemic patients, Kremastinos et al. [30] did not find any significant correlation between the number of blood units transfused and the various echocardiographic indices of left ventricular function. This led the authors to suggest that iron overload is not a critical, but only an additional factor for the development of heart failure, and that viral infections inducing a disorder of cellular immunity could lead to myocardial compromise.

Summary

In this review functional abnormalities of the various organs in β-thalassemia as manifested on liver, spleen, bone marrow, bone and heart scintigraphy are described. Everyone of the above-mentioned modalities reveals a range of scintigraphic patterns depending on the degree of involvement of the organ and the status of maintenance of the patient. In conclusion, Nuclear Medicine offers an alternative imaging approach in β-thalassemia with emphasis on the functional aspect.

Acknowledgements. I wish to thank Dr. C. Politis and Dr. A.B. Mandalaki for referring patients to us for this type of investigation and Professor C. Koutoulidis for giving me permission to use the facilities of the Nuclear Medicine Department of Veterans Administration Hospital "NIMTS" 10 Monis Petraki, Athens, Greece.

References

1. Agnello D, Bruno R, Malizia R, Volpe FP, Lo Iacono F (1985) Ecografia e scintigrafia epatica e splenica in soggetti β-thalassemici politrasfusi. Minerva Pediatr 37: 587–592
2. Ask-Upmark E (1945) Tumour simulating intrathoracic heterotopia of bone marrow. Acta Radiol 26: 425–440

a

b

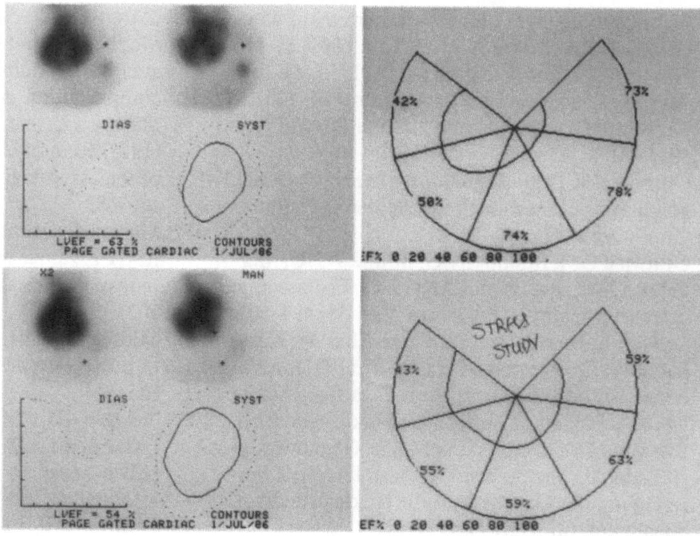

Fig. 7 a, b. Radionuclide ventriculograms of a 20-year-old thalassemic male. **a** A good left ventricular function is manifested at rest (left ventricular ejection fraction (LVEF) = 63%). **b** On ergometric stress, there is significant deterioration of left ventricular performance (LVEF = 54%). Note deterioration of regional EF in the lateral and inferoapical segments, as seen on the regional wall motion image (*right*). (Courtesy of Associate Professor P. Kostamis and Dr. D. T. Kremastinos - Alexandra and Genikon Kratikon Hospitals, Athens)

3. Baker DH (1964) Roentgen manifestations of Cooley's anemia. Ann NY Acad Sci 119: 641–661
4. Beard ME, Necheles TF, Allen DM (1969) Clinical experience with intensive transfusion therapy in Cooley's anemia. Ann NY Acad Sci 165: 415–522
5. Bronn LJ, Paquelet JR, Tetalman MR (1980) Intrathoracic extramedullary hematopoiesis: appearance on 99m Tc-sulphur colloid marrow scan. AJR 134: 1254–1255
6. Caffey J (1957) Cooley's anemia: a review of roentgenographic findings in the skeleton. AJR 78: 381–391
7. Charache S, Page DL (1967) Infarction of bone marrow in the sickle cell disorders. Ann Intern Med 67: 1195–1200
8. Choremis C, Liakakos D, Tseshi C, Moschovakis C (1965) Pathogenesis of osseous lesions in thalassemia. J Pediatr 66: 962–963
9. Datz FL, Taylor A (1985) The clinical use of radionuclide bone marrow imaging. Semin Nucl Med 15: 239–259
10. Dines DM, Canale VC, Arnold WD (1976) Fractures in thalassemia. J Bone Joint Surg (Am) 58: 662–666
11. Doury P (1970) Osteoarthritis and osteitis with multiple foci in the course of septicemia due to salmonella reading complicating thalasso-drepanocytosis. (Fr) Rev Rhum 37: 359-366
12. Ehlers KH, Levin AR, Klein AA, Markensen AL, O'Loughlin JE Jr, Engle MA (1981) The cardiac manifestations of thalassemia major; natural history, noninvasive cardiac diagnostic studies and results of cardiac catheterization. In Engle, Pediatric Cardiovascular Disease, Cardiovasc Clin vol 2, Davis, Philadelphia pp 176-186
13. Engelhard D, Cividalli G, Rachmilewitz EA (1975) Splenectomy in homozygous beta thalassemia: a retrospective study of 30 patients. Br J Haematol 31: 391–402
14. Engle MA (1964) Cardiac involvement in Cooley's anemia. Ann NY Acad Sci 119: 694–702
15. Engle MA, Erlandson M, Smith CH (1964) Late cardiac complications of chronic, severe, refractory anemia with hemochromatosis. Circulation 30: 698–705
16. Exarchou E, Politis C, Vretos E, Pasparakis D, Doganis A, Caramerou A (1981) Fractures and epiphyseal deformities in beta-thalassemia (Gr) Ellén Heirourg Orthop 32: 217–223
17. Fordham EW, Ali A (1981) Radionuclide imaging of bone marrow. Semin Hematol 18: 222–239
18. Freeman AP, Giles RW, Berdoukas VA, Walsh WF, Choy D, Murray PC (1983) Early left ventricular dysfunction and chelation therapy in thalassemia major. Ann Intern Med 99: 450–454

19. Gabrielle OF (1971) Hypoparathyroidism associated with thalassemia. South Med J 64: 115–116
20. Giraud P, Orsini A, Muratore R (1959) Le foie dans la maladie de Cooley. Pediatrie 14: 125
21. Gordon HW, (1959) Hemopoietine Physiol Rev 39: 1–40
22. Gordon HS (1970) Regulation of hematopoiesis, vol 1. Red cell production. Appleton-Century-Crofts, New York
23. Gratwick GM, Bullough PG, Bohne WHO, Markenson AL, Peterson CM (1978) Thalassemic osteoarthropathy. Ann Intern Med 88: 494–501
24. Gyftaki E, Binopoulos D, Kesse-Elias M, Karakatsanis K, Alevizou-Terzaki V (1971) Liver image studies in homozygous Beta thalassemia by the scintillation camera. In: Nuklearmedizin, Radionuklide in der Hämatologie. Gegenwärtiger Stand der Therapie mit Radionukliden. 9. Jahrestagung der Gesellschaft für Nuklearmedizin. Schattauer, Stuttgart
25. Henry WL, Nienhuis AW, Weiner M et al. (1978) Echocardiographic abnormalities in patients with transfusion-dependent anemia and secondary myocardial iron deposition. Am J Med 64: 547–555
26. Hewstone AS, Davidson GP (1972) Yersinia enterocolitica septicaemia with arthritis in a thalassaemic child. Med J Aust 1: 1035–1038
27. Karpathios TH (1978) Abrupt spleen size changes in homozygous β-thalassemia. Thesis, University of Athens, Athens.
28. Karpathios TH, Antypas A, Dimitriou P, Nicolaidou P, Fretzayas A, Thomaidis T, Matsaniotis N (1982) Spleen size changes in children with homozygous β-thalassemia in relation to blood transfusion. Scand J Haematol 28: 220–226
29. Knoblich R (1960) Extramedullary hematopoiesis presenting as intrathoracic tumors: report of a case in a patient with thalassemia minor. Cancer 13: 462–468
30. Kremastinos DT, Toutouzas PK, Vyssoulis GP, Venetis CA, Avgoustakis DG (1984) Iron overload and left ventricular performance in β-thalassemia. Acta Cardiologica 39: 29–40
31. Leon MB, Borer JS, Bacharach SL, Green MV, Benz EJ, Griffith P, Nienhuis AW (1979) Detection of early cardiac dysfunction in patients with severe beta-thalassemia and chronic iron overload. N Engl J Med 301: 1143–1148
32. MacDonald RA, Mallory GK (1960) Hemochromatosis and hemosiderosis; study of 211 autopsied cases. Arch Intern Med 105: 686
33. MacDonald RA (1964) Hemochromatosis and hemosiderosis. Thomas, Springfield pp 3, 94, 207
34. Malamos B, Papavasiliou C, Avramidis A (1962) Tumour-simulating intrathoracic extramedullary hemopoiesis: report of a case. Acta Radiol 57: 227-231
35. March HW, Schlyer SM, Schwartz EE (1952) Mediterranean hemopathic syndrome (Cooley's anemia) in adults: study of a family with unusual complications. Am J Med 13: 46–57
36. Masera G, Jean G, Gazzola G, Novakova M (1976) Role of chronic hepatitis in development of thalassemic liver disease. Arch Dis Child 51: 680–685
37. Masera G, Jean G, Conter V, Terzoli S, Mauri RA, Cazzaniga M (1980) Sequential study of liver biopsy in thalassemia. Arch Dis Child 55: 800–802
38. Middlebrook JE (1956) Thalassemia in a family of pure German extraction. N. Engl J Med 255: 815–817
39. Newton KL, McNeely SG, Novick M (1983) Extramedullary hematopoiesis presenting as a pelvic mass in a patient with β-thalassemia intermedia. JAMA 250: 2178–2179
40. O'Brien RT, Pearson HA, Spencer RP (1972) Transfusion induced decrease in spleen size in thalassemia major: documentation by radioisotopic scan. J Pediatr 81: 105–107
41. Oseas RS, Siddiqui AR, Wellman HN (1982) Usefulness of bone marrow imaging in childhood malignancies. J Pediatr 101: 206–209
42. Paik CH, Alavi I, Dunca G, Weiner L (1970) Thalassemia and gouty arthritis. JAMA 213: 296–297
43. Papavasiliou CG (1965) Tumor simulating intrathoracic extramedullary hemopoiesis. Clinical and roentgenologic considerations. AJR 93: 695–702
44. Politis C, Karamerou A, Block MH, Mahmoud LA (1982) Iron and calcium abnormalities in adolescents with beta-thalassemia major. International Congress, ISH-ISBT, Budapest
45. Robinson AE, Rosse WF, Goodrich JK (1968) Intrathoracic extramedullary hematopoiesis: A scan diagnosis. J Nucl Med 9: 416–419
46. Sebes JI, Massie JD, White TJ, Kraus AP (1984) Pelvic extramedullary hematopoiesis. J Nucl Med 25: 209–210
47. Sella EJ, Goodman AH (1973) Arthropathy secondary to transfusion hemochromatosis. J Bone Joint Surg (AM) 55: 1077–1081
48. Stohlman FJr (1962) Erythropoiesis. New Engl J Med 267: 342–348, 392–399
49. Talbott JH (1959) Gout and blood dyscrasias. Medicine (Baltimore) 38: 173–205
50. Tsachalos P (1960) Gout secondary to thalassemia (minor form of Cooley's disease). (Fr) Rev Rhum 27: 414–416
51. Valdez VA, Jacobstein JG (1980) Decreased bone uptake of technetium-99m polyphosphate in thalassemia major. J Nucl Med 21: 47–49
52. Van Dyke D, Shkurkin C, Price D, Yano Y, Anger HO (1967) Differences in distribution of

45. Robinson AE, Rosse WF, Goodrich JK (1968) Intrathoracic extramedullary hematopoiesis: A scan diagnosis. J Nucl Med 9: 416–419
46. Sebes JI, Massie JD, White TJ, Kraus AP (1984) Pelvic extramedullary hematopoiesis. J Nucl Med 25: 209–210
47. Sella EJ, Goodman AH (1973) Arthropathy secondary to transfusion hemochromatosis. J Bone Joint Surg (AM) 55: 1077–1081
48. Stohlman FJr (1962) Erythropoiesis. New Engl J Med 267: 342–348, 392–399
49. Talbott JH (1959) Gout and blood dyscrasias. Medicine (Baltimore) 38: 173–205
50. Tsachalos P (1960) Gout secondary to thalassemia (minor form of Cooley's disease). (Fr) Rev Rhum 27: 414–416
51. Valdez VA, Jacobstein JG (1980) Decreased bone uptake of technetium-99m polyphosphate in thalassemia major. J Nucl Med 21: 47–49
52. Van Dyke D, Shkurkin C, Price D, Yano Y, Anger HO (1967) Differences in distribution of erythropoietic and reticuloendothelial marrow in hematologic disease. Blood 30: 364–374
53. Vierucci A, London WT, Blumberg BS, Sutnick AI, Ragazzini F (1972) Australian antigen and antibody in transfused children with thalassemia. Arch Dis Child 47: 760
54. Wolman IJ (1964) Transfusion therapy in Cooley's anemia. Growth and health as related to long range hemoglobin levels. A progress report. Ann NY Acad Sci 119: 736–747
55. Zaino EC (1980) Pathophysiology of thalassemia. Ann NY Acad Sci 344: 284–304

10 Abdominal Ultrasonography in β-Thalassemia

A. Papanicolaou and N. C. Gourtsoyiannis

Introduction

Children with β-thalassemia transfused and followed up regularly are prone to develop symptoms of iron overload early in life. Parenchymal iron loading, largely in the form of ferritin, results in widespread hemosiderosis, responsible for tissue damage in most of the abdominal organs.

Recent advances in pediatric ultrasonography, on the other hand, can provide highly detailed images of intra-abdominal structures, which can yield a specific and accurate diagnosis [1]. Although other noninvasive modalities, namely magnetic resonance (MR) or dual-energy computed-tomography (CT) scanning can be successfully used in quantification of tissue iron stores [2, 3], abdominal ultrasonography can offer the potential for detection, localization, and accurate assessment of various morphological changes associated with hemosiderosis in the liver, gallbladder, spleen, pancreas, bowel, uterus, ovaries and abdominal lymph nodes. It can also be useful for following up these changes whenever necessary, without exposing the children to ionizing radiation, by replacing other radiological investigations. In this review, the currently expanding role of ultrasonography in thalassemic patients and the specific sonographic appearances seen in each of the above abdominal organs are described.

Gallbladder

Cholelithiasis in children is more prevalent than is commonly appreciated [4]. Contrary to previous reports, hemolytic anemias are implicated as a predisposing factor in only 20%–30% of cases [5, 6]. However, the reported incidence of cholelithiasis in hereditary spherocytosis ranges from 43 % to 66% [7] and in sickle cell disease from 26% to 37% [8–10].

In patients with thalassemia major, only two systematic studies have been conducted to determine the incidence of gallstones. The results indicate that cholelithiasis is less common today (1,6% for patients aged 0–19 years and 3,6% for patients older than 10 years [11]) than it was in the past (12,5% and 23% respectively [12]). The currently used hypertransfusion therapy has been offered as a possible explanation for this decrease, in that it blocks production by the bone marrow of abnormal red cells responsible for increased bilirubin precipitation in the gallbladder [11].

Ultrasound examination of the gallbladder is particularly applicable to children since it does not use ionizing radiation, it requires minimum preparation and cooperation, and its reliability is not influenced by coexisting liver disease, quite frequent in thalassemic patients. Moreover its accuracy in detecting gallstones in children is as high as it is in adults [13].

Gallbladder calculi appear sonographically as discrete, mobile, echogenic foci with distal shadowing. With meticulous technique, stones as small as 2 mm can be displayed. Microlithiasis pattern or sludge consisting of homogeneous, low-intensity, nonshadowing, and gravity-dependent opacities has also been reported in relation to thalassemia major [4]. In our experience, gallstones in thalassemic patients are usually small and multiple, casting acoustic shadowing (Fig. 1). They also tend to be more prevalent in

Fig. 1. a, b. Cholelithiasis in a thalassemic 12-year-old male. Small, discrete gallstones within an enlarged gallbladder. (S, acoustic shadowing.) Numerous, very smal stones casting acoustic shadowing in a 14-year-old female with thalassemia

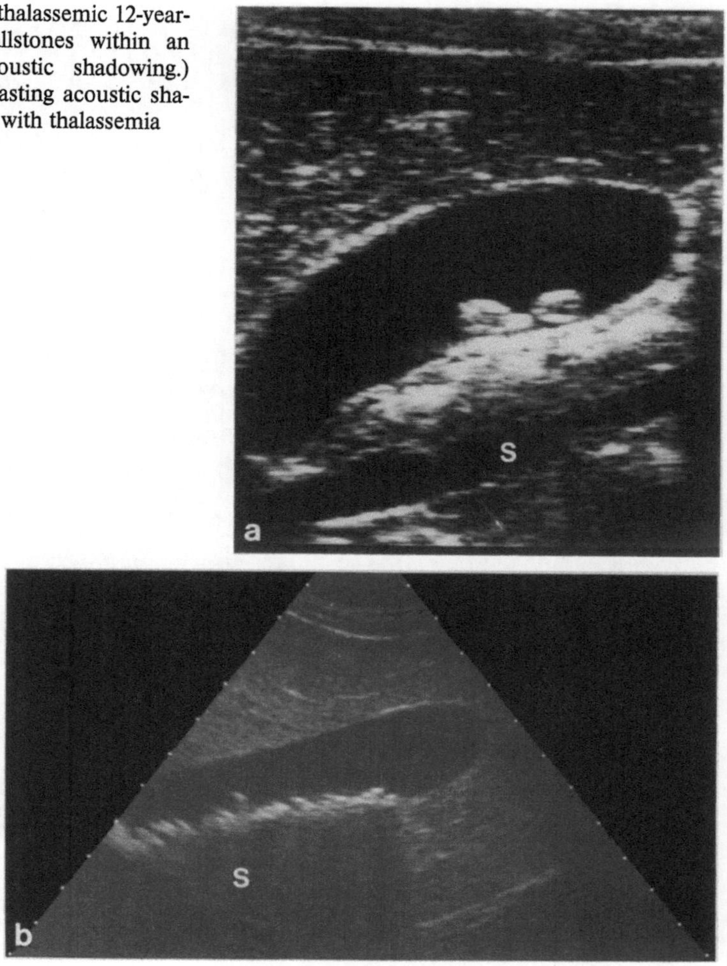

patients with thalassemia intermedia. Hydropic appearance of the pediatric gallbladder represents noninflammatory gallbladder distention, associated with a variety of diseases [14], to which thalassemia has been added recently [11].

Childhood cholecystitis is a relatively rare disease [15, 16]. Although hemolytic anemias are considered particularly prone to develop acalculus cholecystitis [14], this remains to be proved for thalassemic patients. However, enlarged gallbladder with the longest longitudinal diameter exceeding normal limits of the patient's age [17] has been a very frequent feature in our thalassemic patients, even when gallstones were not present.

Infectious hepatitis is considered a relatively common complication of β-thalassemia. In such patients, gallbladder wall thickening may well be an ultrasound finding which represents a nonspecific predictor of cholecystitis in children [18]. Mesenteric adenitis may also be identified sonographically in the same group of patients (Fig. 2).

Liver

Progressive liver damage, due to excessive parenchymal iron loading, occurs remarkably early in the life of thalassemic patients (19). Hepatomegaly and diffusely increased echogenicity of the liver are common, though unspecific, ultrasound features. Liver cirrhosis, secondary to iron overload, is also

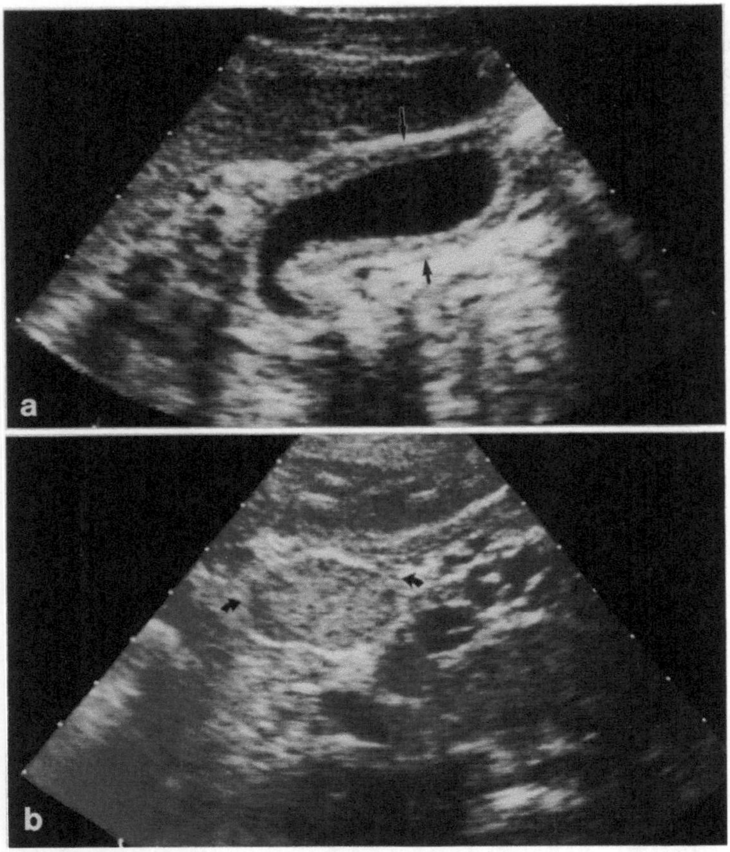

Fig. 2. a Longitudinal left lateral decubitus scan in a 17-year-old thalassemic male with hepatitis, showing marked thickening of the gallbladder wall (*arrows*) without gallstones. **b** Right parasagittal scann in the same patient, showing enlarged lymph node at porta hepatis (*arrows*)

described as a common manifestation in such patients, and it may be followed up by ultrasonography.

Focal liver disease seems quite rare in thalassemia, unlike idiopathic hemochromatosis, where angiomas and hepatomas occur rather frequently [20]. However, liver cell adenoma has been reported in an intensively transfused thalassemic patient, who was under treatment with androgens [21]. Moreover , in a series of 170 thalassemic children followed up by ultrasonography, we also had a case of focal nodular hyperplasia (Fig. 3), which appeared as multiple sharply marginated solid liver nodules of decreased echogenicity, ranging from 1 to 2.3 cm in diameter. Quite recently, on the other hand, the first case of hepatocellular carcinoma in a 22-year-old male, serum and tissue hepatitis B surface antigen (HbsAg7) negative, with thalassemia major was reported [22].

It is fair to assume that the longer survival of thalassemic patients, due to improved transfusion and chelation therapy, will lead to new pathological expressions, in this context. High-resolution ultrasonography is considered as the initial procedure of choise for detection of focal hepatic lesions [23, 24], including such as may appear in patients with thalassemia.

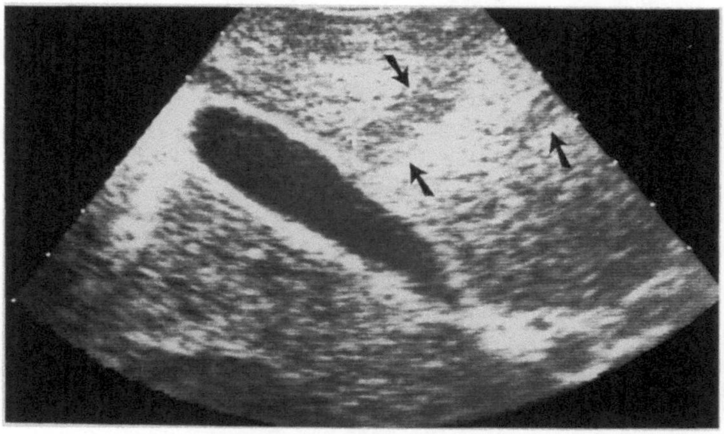

Fig. 3. Focal nodular hyperplasia. Multiple well-defined nodules (*arrows*), slightly less echogenic than the liver, with normal colloid uptake in a 17-year-old female with thalassemia

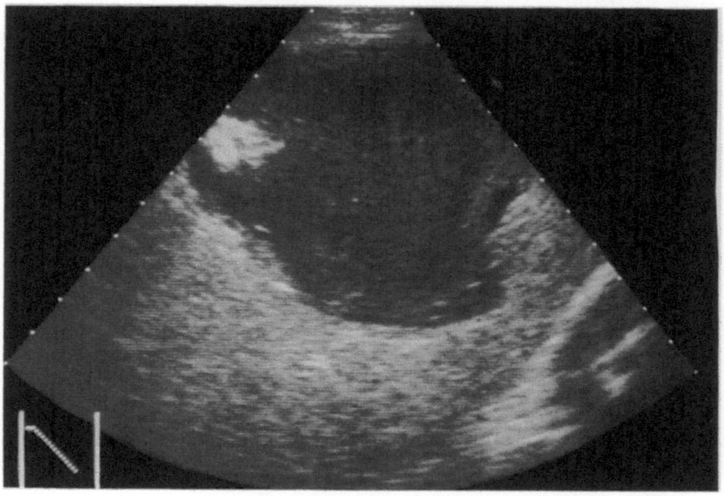

Fig. 4. Splenic abscess. Large, well-defined hypoechoic mass containing scattered echoes in a 13-year-old female thalassemic with septicemia

Spleen

The normal echo texture of the spleen is usually described as fine, uniform, stippled, transonic, and weakly echogenic [25].

Erythropoietic abnormalities generally produce splenomegaly with an isoechoic splenic pattern (same density as the liver) [26].

Diffuse involvement of the spleen in thalassemic patients causes no definite intrasplenic pattern, except for unspecific medium-level echogenicity, presumably secondary to iron deposition within the red pulp. Moderate-to-gross splenomegaly is another very frequent and nonspecific ultrasound finding in this group of patients. In sickle cell anemia, on the contrary, the spleen shrinks, its contour becomes scarred, and its echo texture strongly reflective. Single infarcts, on the other hand, produce well-defined reflective spots in an otherwise uniform echo pattern [27]. Quite rarely, splenic abscesses may also be seen in thalassemic patients, in cases with septicemia (Fig. 4).

Pancreas

Pancreatic insufficiency with frank diabetes mellitus, or at least biochemical evidence of abnormal glucose metabolism, probably

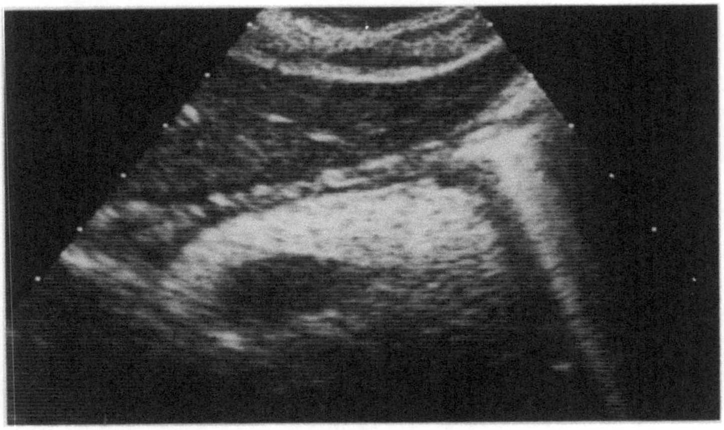

Fig. 5 Diffusely hyperechoic pancreas in an 18-year-old male thalassemic with long-standing diabetes

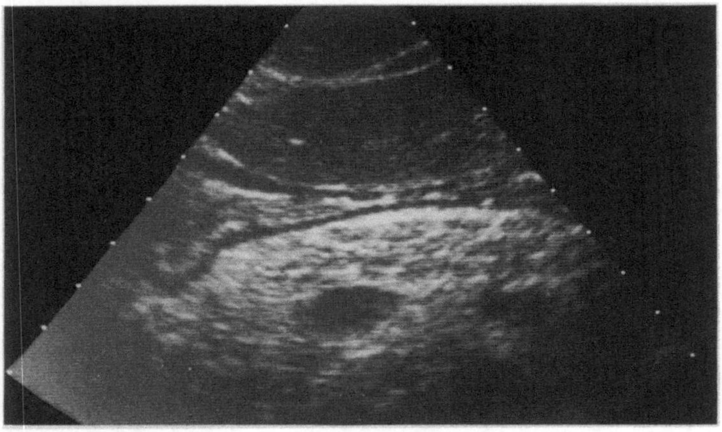

Fig. 6. Echo-dense pattern evenly distributed within the pancreas in a 16-year-old female thalassemic without evidence of diabetes

represents the commonest endocrine abnormality complicating β-thalassemia [19]. In all our β-thalassemic patients with diabetes ultrasonography showed a normal-sized pancreas with grossly increased echogenicity, usually exceeding that of the liver (Fig. 5).

Increased echo texture was also identified in β-thalassemic patients with no clinical evidence of diabetes. Such patients demonstrated varied degrees of sonodense pancreatic patterns, ranging from a discrete net of echogenic areas, distributed within normal pancreatic tissue, to a diffuse parenchymal echogenicity equal to or greater than that of the liver (Fig. 6). In contrast, increased echogenicity of the pancreas was not a feature in our patients with thalassemia intermedia, where regular transfusion was not required.

Ultrasound findings in β-thalassemia are directly associated to the fibrous reaction secondary to iron overload of the pancreas, which is part of the widespread iron deposition including most of the endocrine glands.

So far, there has been no objective correlation between the degree of pancreatic echogenicity and the severity of pancreatic insufficiency or impairment. However, pancreatic sonography may be a useful noninvasive indicator both for assessment of transfusional hemosiderosis and for following chelation therapy [28].

Uterus and Ovaries

Delayed or absent puberty and hypogonadism probably represent the first indi-

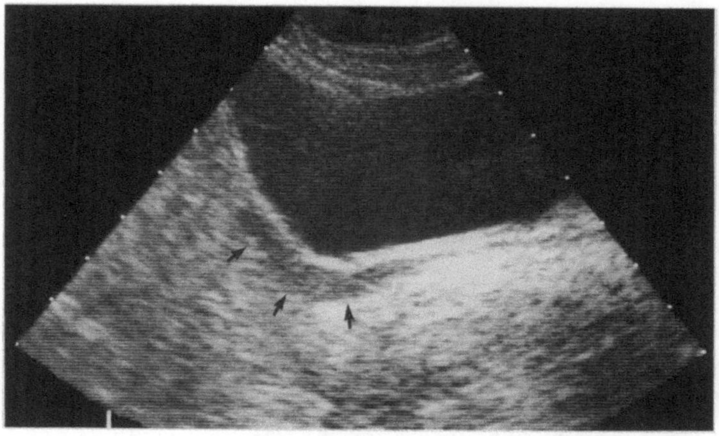

Fig. 7. Tubular appearance of a small, infantile-type uterus (*arrows*), measuring 3.2 x 0.6 cm, in a 24-year-old female with thalassemia

cation of endocrine abnormalities seen in transfusion-dependent thalassemia major. In a recent report failure of pubertal development was observed in more than 50% of such patients over 14 years of age [29]. It is suggested that due to extreme sensitivity to iron toxicity, even small amounts of iron accumulated in the first years of life may produce such irreversible damage to endocrine glands [30].

Pelvic ultrasonography is particularly applicable for assessing ovarian size and structure and uterine changes, as well as following up response to therapy. It can also play a key role in classification and management of disorders of sexual maturation, reducing the need for more complex biochemical measurements [31]. In thalassemic children, the uterus usually exhibits infantile morphology and size on ultrasonography even a long time after the onset of puberty (Fig. 7). The ovaries display a homogeneous, solid ultrasound pattern. Their mean volume seldom exceeds 1,5 cm^3, and they may contain very few small follicles, 2-4 mm in diameter (Fig. 8).

Yersinia Enterocolica Infections

Infection with *Yersinia enterocolica* has a very low incidence in Greece, and only sporadic cases have been documented until recently in otherwise normal individuals [32]. Severe clinical manifestatitons of *Y enterocolitica* infections, such as enteritis, mesenteric adenitits, hepatosplenic abscesses or septicemia, are primarily encountered in immunosuppressed or severely ill patients and in patients with iron overload [33–35].

Alterations in iron metabolism seem to confer increased host susceptibility to a variety of microorganisms [36]. However, *Y. enterocolitica* stands out as one of the most iron-depended of all microbes since systemic infections with this organism are virtually unknown in patients with normal iron stores [37]. This remarkable relationship can be explained by the inability of *Y. enterocolitica* to synthesize iron-binding compounds or siderophores [38].

It is also postulated that increased susceptibility to yersiniosis may be attributable to chelation therapy with desferrioxamine B, and not to iron overload per se [39]. The incidence of *Y. enterocolitica* infections in patients with thalassemia, regularly transfused, can be as high as 11% [40].

A painful palpable mass at the right iliac fossa is one of the most prominent clinical findings, caused by acute terminal ileitis and mesenteric adenitis. Location, measurements, pattern recognition, and clearance of abdominal mass in such patients have recently been followed up by ultrasonography. Sonographic findings are due to a combination of symmetrical, marked thi

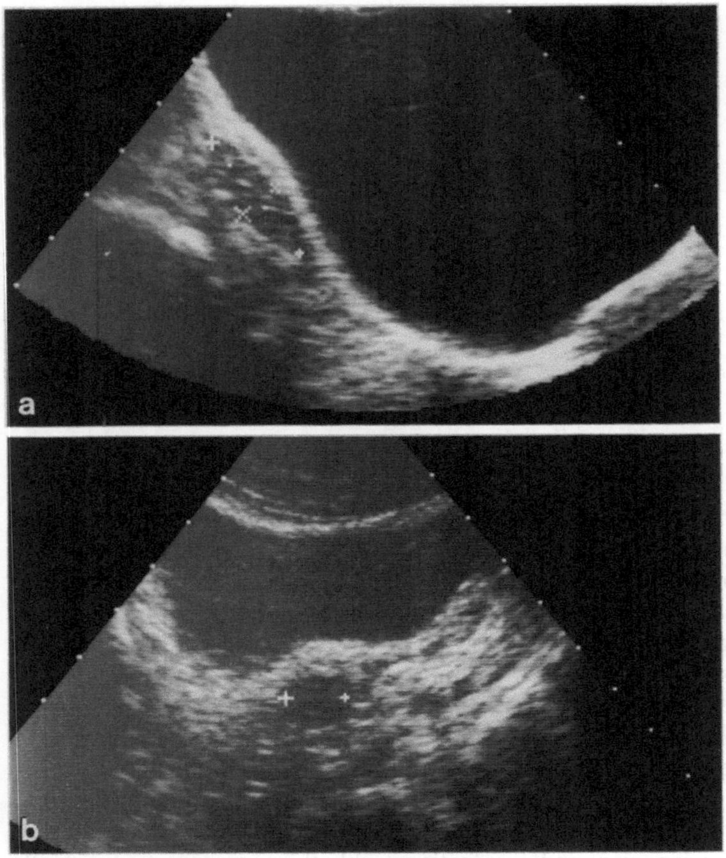

Fig. 8. a Longitudinal scan and **b** transverse scan, showing a small (volume, 0.9 cm^3) left ovary in a 22- year-old female with thalassemia and sexual infantilism

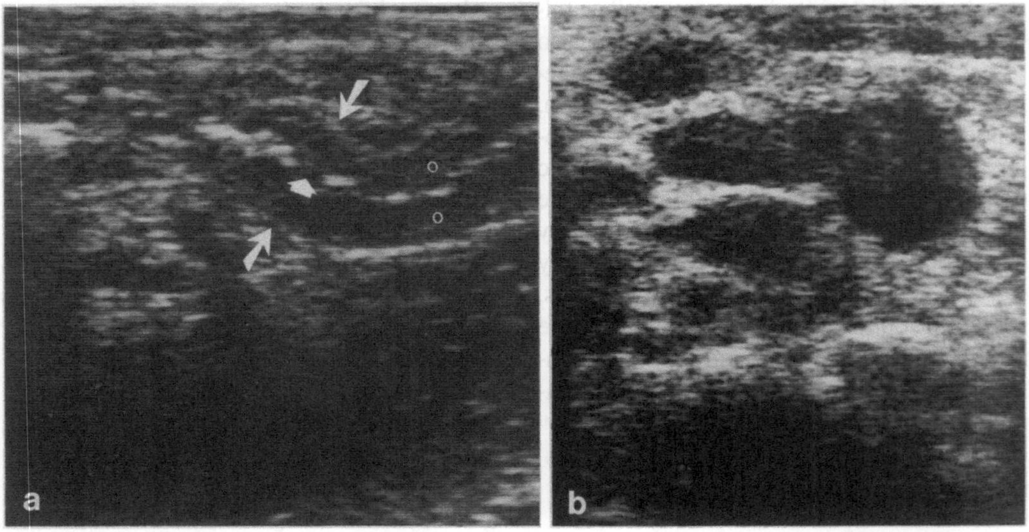

Fig. 9 a, b. *Y. enterocolitica* infection in a 12-year-old male with thalassemia. **a** Longitudinal view of inflamed terminal ileum (*arrows*) with symmetrical wall thickening (o). Broad echogenic lining (*arrowhead*) within echo-poor center represents the obliterated lumen. **b** A group of enlarged mesenteric lymph nodes. Echo-poor nodes are well demarcated from the echogenic surroundings

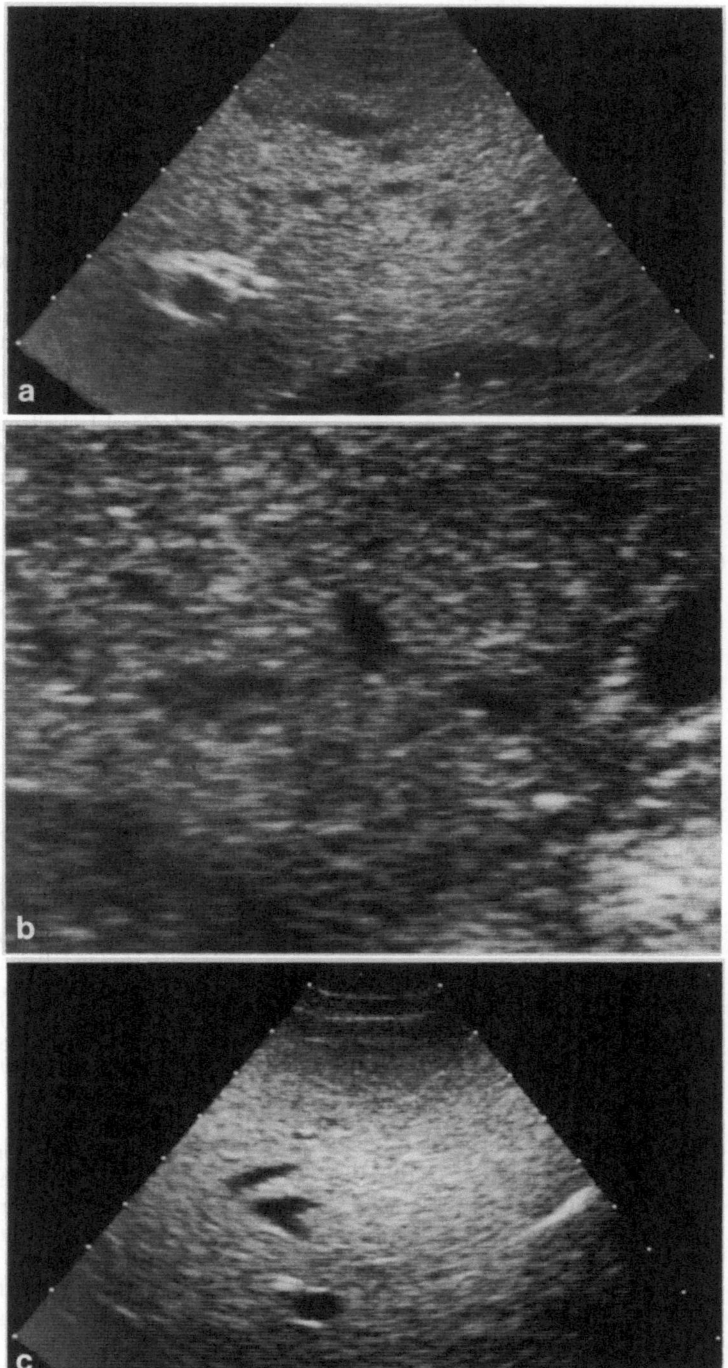

Fig. 10. a Parasagittal scan of right lobe of liver in a 9-year-old male thalassemic with *Y enterocolitica* infection, showing small, ill-defined hypoechoic areas, representing microabscesses. **b** Enlarged oblique view of the same patient, showing microabscesses. **c** Same patient 3 weeks after therapy, showing complete clearance of lesions

ckening of the terminal ileum and enlarged mesenteric lymph nodes. On cross sections perpendicular to the lumen, the terminal ileum will appear as a "donut" or a flattened bull's-eye. On longitudinal views, it will again appear as a tubular structure. The thickened bowel wall, exceeding 1 cm in diameter, appears echopoor, though its lumen with mucus and entrapped gas appears quite echogenic (Fig. 9a).

Enlarged lymph nodes appear ovoid or spherical instead of the normal disclike shape. They are sonolucent and sharply marginated and in most cases they are numerous (Fig. 9b). Their anteroposterior diameter must exceed 5 mm.

The ultrasound appearance of bowel disorders is generally considered nonspecific. Quite a number of infiltrative and inflammatory diseases can cause local thickening of the bowel wall and compromise its lumen [41–43]. In addition, enlarged mesenteric lymph nodes may be found in association with acute appendicitis in about 40% of patients [44]. However with increasing experience, and using real-time ultrasonography, it appears that a characteristic and almost conspicuous pattern recognition of *Y. enterocolitica* terminal ileitis and mesenteric adenitis has emerged [45]. Our experience with 19 thalassemic patients suffering from *Y. enterocolitica* infections indicates that ultrasound findings are extremely valuable in establishing the correct diagnosis, before the results of serologic tests or stool cultures become available. It also indicates that ultrasonography can be very helpful in obviating the need for appendicectomy in patients with *Y. enterocolitica* infections. Additional ultrasound features in thalassemic patients with *Y. enterocolitica* septicemia include small abscesses of the liver or spleen (Fig. 10). Following up each of the above clinical manifestations until complete clearance is another distinct and succesful role for ultrasonography in patients with *Y. enterocolitica* infections.

References

1. Blumhagen JD, Weinberger E (1986) Pediatric gastrointestinal ultrasonography. In: Sanders RC, Hill M (eds.) Ultrasound annual 1986. Raven, New York
2. Goldberg HI, Cann CE, Moss AA, Ohto M, Brito A, Federle M (1982) Noninvasive quantification of liver iron in dogs with hemochromatosis using dual-energy CT scanning. Invest Radiol 17: 375–380
3. Brasch RC, Wesbey GE, Gooding CA, Koerper MA (1984) Magnetic resonance imaging of transfusional hemosiderosis complicating thalassemia major. Radiology 150: 767–771
4. Garel L, Lallemand D, Montagne JP, Forel F, Sauvegrain J (1981) The changing aspects of cholelithiasis in children through a sonographic study. Pediatr Radiol 11: 75–79
5. Harned RK, Babitt DR (1975) Cholelithiasis in children. Radiology 117: 391–393
6. Henschke CI, Teele RL (1983) Cholelithiasis in children. Recent observations. J Ultrasound Med 2: 481–484
7. Bates GC, Brown CH (1952) Incidence of gallbladder disease in chronic hemolytic anemia (spherocytosis). Gastroenterology 21: 104–107
8. Lachman BS, Lazerson J, Starshak RJ, Vaughters FM, Werlin SL (1979) The prevalence of cholelithiasis in sickle cell disease as diagnosed by ultrasound and cholecystography. Pediatrics 64: 601–603
9. Sarnail S, Slovis TL, Corbett DP, Emami A, Whitten CF (1980) Incidence of cholelithiasis in sickle cell anemia using the ultrasonic gray-scale technique. Pediatrics 96: 1005–1008
10. Pennels MB, Dunne MG, Grossman NJ, Schwartz AD (1984) Cholelithiasis in patients with major sickle hemoglobinopathies. Am J Dis Child 138: 66–67
11. Borgna-Pignatti C, de Stefano P, Pajno D, Tomasi G, Gatti C (1981) Cholelithiasis in children with thalassemia major. An ultrasonographic study. J Pediatr 99: 243–244
12. Dewey KW, Grossman H, Canale VC (1970) Cholelithiasis in thalassemia major. Radiology 96: 385–388
13. Buschi AJ, Norman A, Brenbridge AG (1980) Sonographic diagnosis of cholelithiasis in childhood. Am J Dis Child 134: 575–576
14. Durell CA, Vincent LM, Mittelstaedt CA (1984) Gallbladder ultrasonography in clinical context. Semin Ultrasound 5: 315–332
15. Kumari S, Lee WJ, Baron MG (1979) Hydrops of the gallbladder in a child: diagnosis by ultrasonography. Pediatrics 63: 295–297
16. Greenberg M, Kangarloo H, Cochran ST et al.

(1980) The ultrasonographic diagnosis of cholecystitis and cholelithiasis in children. Radiology 137: 745-749
17. Slovis TL, Hight DW, Philippart AJ, Dubois RS (1980) Sonography in the diagnosis and management of hydrops of the gallbladder in children with mucocutaneous lymph node syndrome. Pediatrics 65: 789-794
18. Patriquin HB, di Pietro M, Barber FE, Teel RL (1983) Sonography of thickened gallbladder wall: causes in children. AJR 141: 57-60
19. Weatherall DJ, Clegg JB (eds.) (1981) The β-thalassemias. In: The thalassemia syndromes. Blackwell Scientific, Oxford, p 157
20. Milder MS, Cook JD, Stray S, Finch C (1980) Idiopathic hemochromatosis, an interim report. Medicine (Baltimore) 59: 34-49
21. Potter B (1982) Ultrasound. In: Franken EAJr (eds.) Gastrointestinal imaging in pediatrics. Harper and Row, Philadelphia, p 608
22. Borgna-Pignatti C, de Stefano P, Sessa F, Avato F (1986) Hepatocellular carcinoma in thalassemia major. Med Pediatr Oncol 14: 326-328
23. Bernardino ME, Sones PJ Jr, Price RB, Berkman WA (1984) Coordinated diagnostic imaging. In: Simeone J (ed.) Clinics in diagnostic ultrasound, vol. 14. Churchill Livingstone, New York, pp 221-234
24. Holm J, Jacobsen B (1986) Accuracy of dynamic ultrasonography in the diagnosis of malignant liver lesions. J Ultrasound Med 5: 1-4
25. Tayler KJW, Milan J (1976) Differential diagnosis of chronic splenomegaly by gray-scale ultrasonography: clinical observations and digital A-scan analysis. Br J Radiol 49: 519-525
26. Mittelstaedt CA, Partain CL (1980) Ultrasonic-pathologic classification of splenic abnormalities: gray-scale patterns. Radiology 134: 697-705
27. Cosgrove DO, McGready RV (1982) Ultrasound imaging: liver - spleen - pancreas. Wiley, Chichester, p 344
28. Erttman R, Hausdorf G, Landbeck G (1983) Pancreatic sonography in thalassemia major. Clin Pediatr (Phila.) 195: 97-99
29. de Sanctis V, Tanas R, Borgatti L, Vullo C, Bagni B (1987) Endocrine complications in thalassemia major. In: Sirchia G and Zanella A (eds.) Thalassemia today. Centro Transfusionale, Ospedale Maggiore Policlinico di Milano, Milan, pp93-98
30. Borgna-Pignatti C, de Stefano P, Zonta L, Vullo C, de Sanctis V, Melevendi C, Naselli A, Masera G, Terzoli S, Gabbutti V, Piga A (1985) Growth and sexual maturation in thalassemia major. J Pediatr 106: 150-155
31. Stanhop R, Adams J, Jacobs HS, Brook CGD (1985) Ovarian ultrasound assessment in normal children, idiopathic precocious puberty and during low dose pulsatile gonadotropin releasing hormone treatment of hypogonadotrophic hypogonadism. Arch Dis Child 60: 116-119
32. Maniatis A (1982) *Yersinia enterocolitica* infections (yersiniosis). Iatriki 41: 123-132
33. Kohl S (1979) *Yersinia enterocolitica* infection in children. Pediatr Clin North Am 26: 433-443
34. Bouza E, Dominguer A, Meseguer M, Buron L, Boixeda D, Revillo M, Rafael L, Martinez-Beltran J (1980) *Yersinia enterocolitica* septicemia. J Pediatr 74: 404-409
35. Shapiro E (1981) *Yersinia enterocolitica* septicemia in normal infants. Am J Dis Child 135: 477-478
36. Finkelstein RA, Sciortino CV, McIntosh MA (1983) Role of iron in microbe-host interactions. Rev Infect Dis 5: 759-777
37. Robins-Browne RM, Rabson AR, and Koornhof HJ (1979) Generalized infection with *Yersinia enterocolitica* and the role of iron. Contrib Microbiol Immunol 5: 277-282
38. Perry RD, Brubaker RR (1979) Accumulation of iron by yersiniae. J Bacteriol 137: 1290-1298
39. Robins-Browne RM, Pripic JK (1983) Desferrioxamine and systemic yersiniosis. Lancetii 1372
40. Kattamis C, Ladis V, Vekiou-Samara A (1985) *Yersinia enterocolitica* infection in patients with β- thalassemia. 2nd Mediterraneann Meeting on Thalassemia, "Milanomedicina '85", Milan, 28-30 November 1985
41. Yeh HC Rabinowitz JG (1982) Ultrasonography of gastrointestinal tract. Semin Ultrasound 331: 347
42. Dubbins PA (1984) Ultrasound demonstration of bowel wall thickness in inflammatory bowel disease. Clin Radiol 35: 227-231
43. Miller JH, Kamberling CR (1984) Ultrasound scanning of the gastrointestinal tract in children: subject review. Radiology 152: 671-677
44. Puylaert JBCM (1986) Acute appendicitis: US evaluation using graded compression. Radiology 158: 355-360
45. Puylaert JBCM (1986) Mesenteric adenitis and acute terminal ileitis: US evaluation using graded compression. Radiology 161: 691-695

11 Cardiac Complications in Thalassemia Syndromes: Clinical and Radiological Considerations

A. C. Papaioannou and S. Antoniadis

Introduction

Cardiac complications frequently associated with endocrinopathies and infections are the most common cause of morbidity and death in patients with homozygous thalassemia syndromes. In many cases, symptoms of heart lesions may appear in early childhood, but death usually occurs during the 2nd or 3rd decade [14–16]. Early diagnosis and treatment of cardiac complications in this disease are essential for the survival of these patients [40].

In Greece, thalassemia syndromes have a high prevalence, ranging from 5% to 15% in the different geographic areas of the country, and constitute a major social and public health problem [34–36, 46, 51, 53].

Pathophysiology and Clinical Course

Cardiac involvement has long been known to accompany anemia and depends on the latter's severity and duration. The pathophysiological mechanisms which cause the heart complications are not yet fully understood. In severe chronic anemia, the low level of hemoglobin (Hb) reduces the capacity of the blood to transport sufficient oxygen to the tissues. It has been shown that when Hb falls below 7 g/100 ml, cardiac output increases, even at rest, in order to supply the requirements of oxygen to the tissues [4, 7, 12, 55]. The main factors involved in the elevation of cardiac output are alterations in ventricular preload, ventricular contractility, and ventricular afterload. Decreased ventricular afterload is probably the most important cause of high cardiac output [33]. Hypoxia of the tissues generates several counterbalancing mechanisms, resulting in peripheral vasodilatation, increased arteriovenous shunts, and reduction of systemic vascular resistance [3]. Lowered viscosity of the blood also plays an important role [23].

These observations support the view that the increase of cardiac output is due primarily to the increase of contractility and stroke volume of the left ventricle and secondarily to the heart rate [50]. The contractility of the left ventricle increases when ventricular afterload decreases and the viscosity of the blood is low.

Under these circumstances, ventricular function is preserved until some stage of the disease when gradually or abruptly the ventricular muscle loses its ability to contract efficiently. High cardiac output and the damage to the heart muscle produced by hypoxia are the main causes of the appearance of terminal heart failure [11, 55]. This type of heart failure differs from classical congestive heart failure.

In thalassemia, ventricular function is additionally impaired by the deposition of iron in the heart muscle. Often, it is difficult to determine whether the appearance of heart failure results primarily from anemia or the presence of hemosiderosis [6, 8].

The accumulation of iron in tissues – notably the heart, liver, pancreas, and endocrine glands – may also lead to fibrosis, permanent damage, and varying degrees of dysfunction of these organs. In fact, at autopsy a widespread iron deposition and fibrosis of the tissues are found [1, 6, 45, 49, 52].

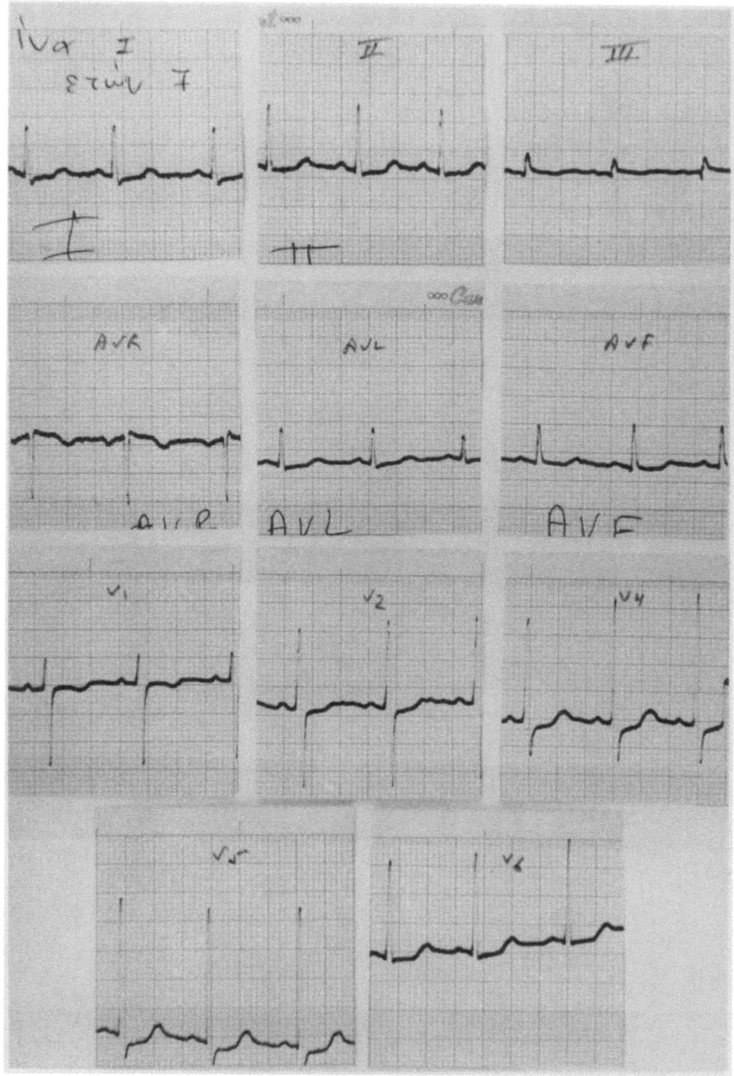

Fig. 1. Electrocardiogram (ECG) of a thalassemic 8-year-old female, showing left ventricular predominance and slight depression of ST segment in V_5–V_6

The clinical course in patients suffering from thalassemia varies. They are usually asymptomatic during infancy and early childhood. Cardiovascular symptoms usually appear in later childhood [14, 16, 39]. Their severity and progress depend on the severity of anemia, method of treatment, and degree of hemosiderosis. When the cardiac lesions have progressed, symptoms and signs of frank heart failure, such as orthopnea, tachycardia, venous distention, hepatomegaly, and pitting edema, are evident.

On auscultation, a third or fourth heart sound is frequently audible over the apical area. There is no murmur that could not be caused by severe anemia [28, 30]. Occasionally, middiastolic murmurs or rumble can be heard over the areas of the mitral, tricuspid, or aortic valves. We have documented in many instances the presence of murmurs suggestive of mitral stenosis, which disappeared immediately after a blood transfusion.

Arrhythmias are frequently encountered and in some cases may be bizarre. The elec-

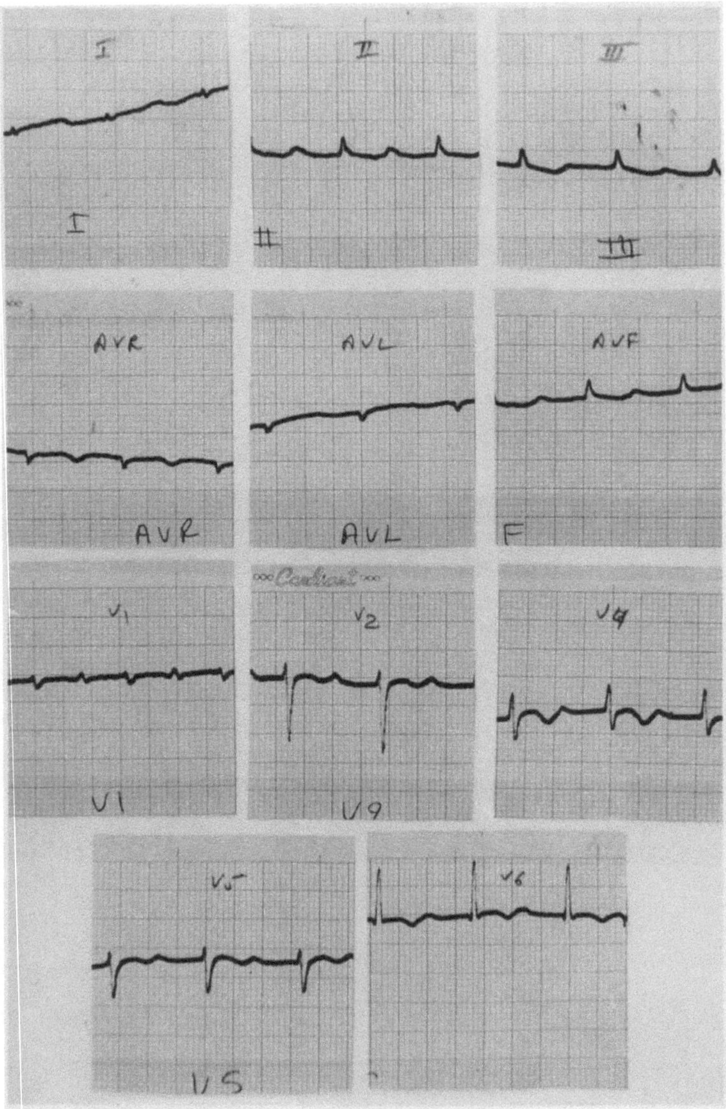

Fig. 2. ECG changes compatible with myopericarditis

trocardiogram helps in determining the type of arrhythmia, ventricular hypertrophy, and ischemia, and also ectopic impulse formation and conduction disorders (Figs. 1, 2).

Pericarditis is not an uncommon complication. It may be preceded by fever of unknown origin or acute precordial pain referring to the shoulder. A friction rub or sterile pericardial effusion frequently accompany attacks of pericarditis.

Heart failure occurs gradually or suddenly after exacerbation of anemia or acute infection. When symptoms and signs of frank heart failure appear, a life expectancy of more than 2 years is exceptional.

Treatment depends mainly on regular blood transfusions. New regimens of transfusion and removal of iron by various chelation agents have considerably improved the clinical picture of the disease [2, 9, 10, 35, 37, 47, 48]. However, a method has not yet been found that would be sufficiently effective in

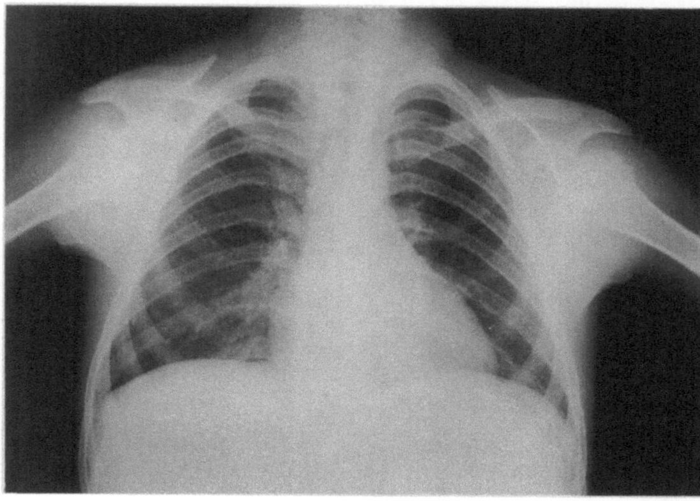

Fig. 3. Chest X-ray film of a thalassemic 3-year-old male, showing normal cardiac shadow

curing anemia, preventing iron deposition, and changing the overall prognosis of the disease [14].

The appearance of congestive heart failure needs prompt and careful management. Digitalis should be used carefully because the iron-loaded myocardium is very sensitive. Diuretics, restriction of salt, and bed rest are parts of the therapeutic regimen. Unfortunately, when heart failure appears, the treatment has only a temporary effect. Associated angina pectoris can be relieved effectively by vasodilators or beta-blockers.

In serious types of arrhythmias, digoxin or special antiarrhythmic drugs can be used. It should be kept in mind that bizarre arrhythmias may lead to sudden death.

The treatment of pericarditis consists of low-salt diet, diuretics, administration of antibiotics to prevent infection, and therapy for heart failure, if present. According to our experience, the use of low doses of cortisone for 1 week is helpful. Pericarditis usually lasts for 1 week and has a benign course; however, recurrences have been observed not infrequently. Occasionally, such cases are complicated by tamponade, in which case pericardiotomy is necessary.

One important aspect in the treatment of thalassemia, which has only been emphasized recently, is the need for psychological support of these patients. These children are loaded not only with iron but also with fear and anxiety, and they always need special guidance and sexual and professional orientation. It is a tragic irony that their "iron hearts" are so fragile both literally and metaphorically. There is hope that newer and more radical methods for the treatment of thalassemia will be applied in the near future.

Radiological and Echocardiographic Imaging of the Heart

Roentgenography of the chest is a simple and reliable method for estimation of heart size. In early childhood, the heart may appear normal (Fig. 3). Later, follow-up by chest roentgenography may show progressive enlargement of the heart, particularly of the left ventricle (Fig. 4). In some patients treated regularly with blood transfusions, the heart may be normal-sized or slightly enlarged even at an older age (Fig. 5). In patients with cardiac involvement or pericarditis, there is marked cardiomegaly and pulmonary vascular markings suggestive of congestive heart failure (Fig. 6).

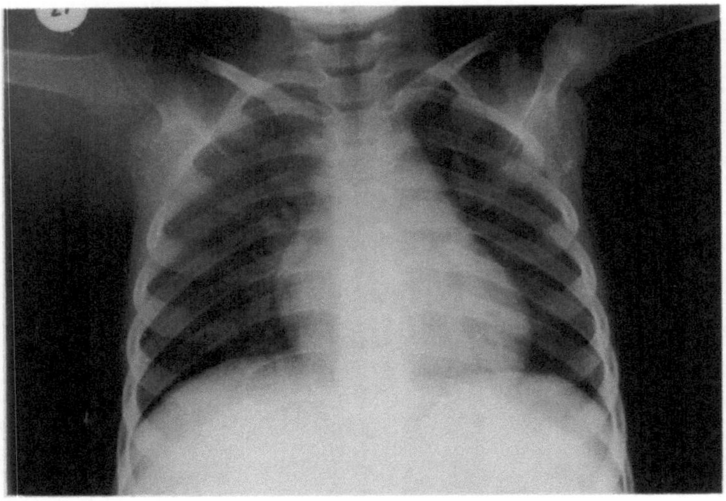

Fig. 4. Chest X-ray film of a thalassemic 7-year-old female, showing slight enlargement of the heart and left ventricle

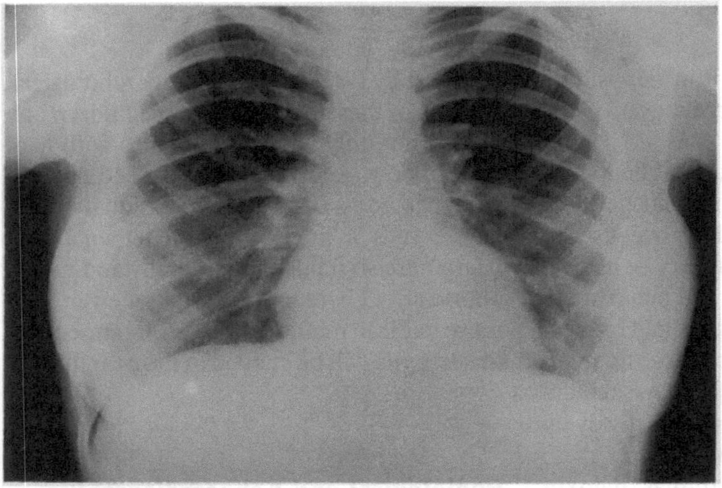

Fig. 5. Chest X-ray film of a thalassemic 20-year-old female, regularly transfused. The heart size at this age is still within normal limits

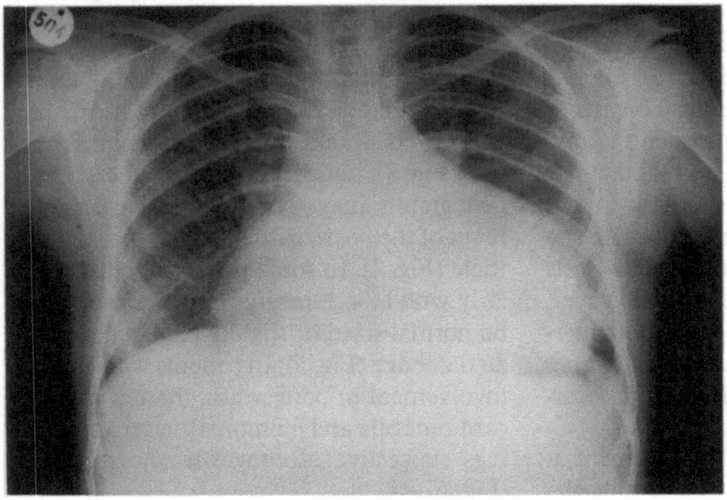

Fig. 6. Chest X-ray film of a thalassemic 15-year-old female, showing considerable increase in heart size due to pericarditis

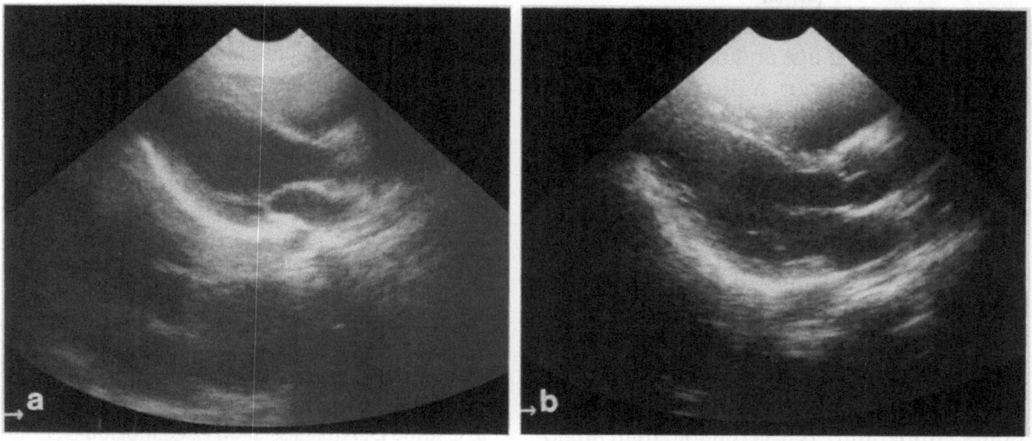

Fig. 7 a, b. Echocardiograms of a thalassemic 10-year-old female, showing mild dilatation of the left ventricle with normal contractility

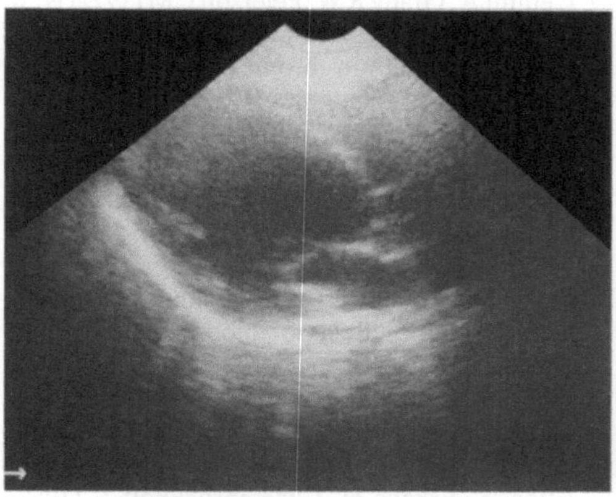

Fig. 8. Echocardiogram of a thalassemic 12-year-old female, showing dilatation of the left ventricle with decreased contractility

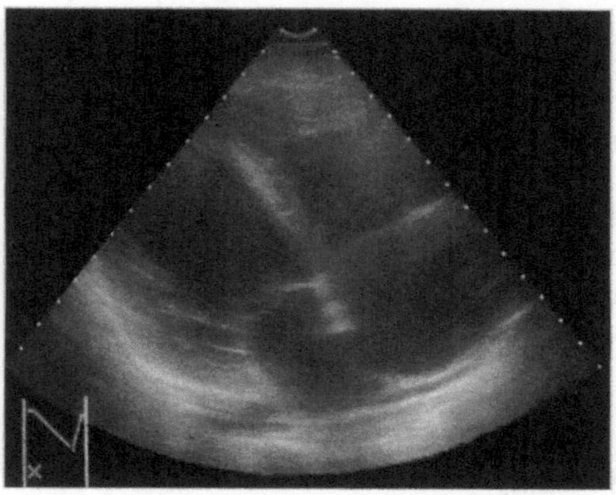

Fig. 9. Echocardiogram of a thalassemic 20-year-old male complicated with diabetes. There is dilatation of all cardiac chambers, especially the left ventricle, and poor contractility. This patient died a few days later

Echocardiography is today the diagnostic method of choice for evaluation of early and late changes of the morphology and function of the heart. These studies include measurement of ventricular dimensions, wall movement of the heart, and the condition in the pericardium. Estimation of the above parameters by echocardiography also helps in assessing the efficacy of multiple transfusions and the results of chelation therapy [17, 20–22, 25, 26, 31, 32].

Investigations by echocardiography have demonstrated gradual changes of the elliptical shape of the left ventricle during the systole to a more spherical shape maintained during the whole cardiac cycle [54]. In thalassemia, the ventricular wall at an early stage is dilated and thin, and later it is hypertrophied. The internal echo dimensions of the left ventricle in late systole and diastole, as well as those of the right ventricle, left atrium, and aortic root, were found to be increased compared with the values expected for normal children of similar age and body surface [25]. Initially, the posterior wall of the ventricle and the interventricular septum were found to be thinner than expected. The septum in some cases shows an abnormal movement, particularly during systole [54]. In rare instances, the morphological changes of the left ventricle resemble those of constrictive myocardiopathy [5, 38].

Heart catheterization and angiocardiography correlated with echocardiography may complete the cardiac evaluation [18, 29]. Echocardiography is less reliable than angiocardiography and heart catheterization in estimating the stroke volume, cardiac output, pressures in the cardiac chambers, and ejection fraction of the left ventricle [42–44]. For practical purposes, however, two-dimensional echocardiography alone is satisfactory and resolves most of the diagnostic problems (Figs. 7–9). Another advantage of echocardiography over the previously mentioned methods is that is can be repeated frequently and safely without the potential risk of invasive methods.

Summary

Cardiac complications in thalassemia syndromes have been described. Heart involvement is the most common cause of death in these patients. The clinical symptoms, pathophysiology, and laboratory findings have been discussed. The role of radiology, particularly of echocardiography, in establishing the diagnosis of heart involvement has been emphasized. Early diagnosis and treatment of thalassemia considerably improve the clinical course of the disease.

References

1. Anderson WAD, Kissane JM (1977) Pathology, 7th edn. Mosby, Saint Louis
2. Barry M, Flynn MD, Letsky EA, Risdon RA (1974) Long-term chelation therapy in thalassemia major: effect on liver iron concentration. liver histology and clinical progress. Br Med J 2: 16
3. Berne RM (1964) Metabolic regulation of blood flow. Circ Res 15 (suppl 1): 261
4. Brannon ES, Merrill AJ, Warren JV, Stead EA, JR (1945) The cardiac output in patients with chronic anemia as measured by the technic of right atrial catheterization. J Clin Invest 24: 332
5. Brawnwald E (1980) Heart disease. A textbook of cardiovascular medicine. Saunders, Philadelphia
6. Buja LM, Roberts WC (1971) Iron in the heart. Am J Med 51: 209
7. Castle WB, Minot GR (1936) Pathological physiology and clinical description of the anemias. Oxford University Press, New York p 2
8. Catriou D, Athanassiadou E, Gianoglou G, Louridas J, Karatza E, Sklavounou-Tsouroutzoglou S (1985) Chelation therapy and cardiac function in patients with β-thalassemia. Pediatriki 48: 289
9. Cerami A, Grady RW, Peterson CM (1977) New iron chelators. In Zaino EC, Roberts R (eds) Chelation therapy in chronic iron overload. Symposia, Miami
10. Cooper B, Franklin Bunn H, Propper RD, Nathan DG, Rosenthal DS, Moloney WC (1977) Treatment of iron overload in adults with continuous parenteral desferrioxamine. Am J Med 63: 969
11. Duke M, Herbert VD, Abelmann WH (1964) Hemodynamic effects of blood transfusion in chronic anemia. N Engl J Med 271: 975
12. Duke M, Abelmann WH (1969) The hemodynamic response to chronic anemia. Circulation 39: 503
13. Effect S, Erkens H, Grossebrockhoff F (1957) Ultrasonic echo method in cardiological diagnosis. Ger Med Methods 2:325
14. Ehlers KH, Levin AR, Markenson AL, Marcus JR, Klein AA, Hilgartner MW, Engle MA (1980) Longitudinal study of cardiac function in thalassemia major. Ann NY Acad Sci 344: 397
15. Engle MA (1964) Cardiac involvement in Coolley's anemia. Ann NY Acad Sci 119: 694
16. Engle MA, Erlandson M, Smith CH (1967) Late cardiac complications of chronic severe refractory anemia with hemochromatosis. Circulation 30: 698
17. Feigenbaum H, Waldhausen JA, Hyde LP (1965) Ultrasound diagnosis of pericardial effusion. JAMA 191: 107
18. Feigenbaum H, Popp RL, Wolfe SB, et al. (1972) Ultrasound measurements of the left ventricle: a correlation study with angiography. Arch Intern Med 129: 461
19. Feigenbaum H (1981) Echocardiography, 3rd edn. Lea and Febiger, Philadelphia
20. Flynn DM, Hussain MAM, Mitchell A, Myers A,

Gorman A, Hoffbrand AV (1980) Echocardiographic measurements of the left ventricular internal dimension in diastole, in regularly transfused thalassemic children and its correlation with units of blood transfused and age. Proc world pediatric congress, London 1980
21. Fonzo R, Meloni L, de Virgilis S, Turgo M, Raffo M, Cherchi A (1979) Echocardiographic findings in thalassemia major in childhood. Bull Int Card Soc 25: 193
22. Fortuin NJ, Hood WP, Sherman ME, et al. (1971) Determination of left ventricular volumes by ultrasound. Circulation 44: 575
23. Fowler NO, Holmes JC (1975) Blood viscosity and cardiac output in acute experimental anemia. J Appl Physiol 39: 453
24. Fowler NO, Holmes JC (1971) Ventricular function in anemia. J Appl Physiol 31:260
25. Galanis C (1984) Cardiopathy in β-Mediterranean disease. Echocardiographic study. Thesis, University of Athens, Athens
26. Gibson DG (1973) Estimation of left ventricular size by echocardiography. Br Heart J 35: 128
27. Graettinger JS, Parsons RL, Campbell JA (1963) A correlation of clinical and hemodynamic studies in patients with mild and severe anemia with and without congestive failure. Ann Intern Med 58: 617
28. Graham G, Rossi G (1980) Heart disease in infants and children. Arnold, London
29. Grossman W (1976) Cardiac catheterization and angiography Lea and Febiger, Philadelphia
30. Harris TN, Friedman S, Tuncali MT, Hallidi-Smith K (1964) Comparison of innocent murmurs of childhood with cardiac murmurs in high output states. Pediatrics 33: 341
31. Henry WL, Nienhuis AW, Wiener W, Miller DR, Canale VC, Piomelli S (1978) Echocardiography abnormalities in patients with transfusion-dependent anemia and secondary myocardial iron deposition. Am J Med 64: 547
32. Henry WL, Gardin JM, Ware JH (1980) Echocardiographic measurements in normal subjects from infancy to old age. Circulation 62: 1054
33. Hurst J (1986) The heart. McGraw-Hill, New York
34. Kanavakis E, Tzotos S. Liapaki A, Metaxotou-Mavromati A, Kattamis C (1986) Frequency of thalassemia in Greece. Am J Hematol 22:255
35. Kattamis C, Karambula C, Metaxotou-Mavromati A, Ladis V, Constantopoulos A (1978) Prevalence of β^- and β^+ thalassemia genes in Greek children with homozygous β-thalassemia. Hemoglobin 2: 29
36. Kattamis C (1982) The child with thalassemia. Bulletin of the Int Ped Assoc 4: 19
37. Kattamis C (1985) Basic principles in the treatment of thalassemia. Bull 1st Ped Clin University of Athens 32: 189
38. Kremastinos DT, Toutouzas PK, Karas SM, Vissoulis GP, Avgoustakis DG (1982) The function and morphology of the left ventricle in homozygous β-thalassemia. Hell Heart Rev 23: 173
39. Kuaku Ohene - Frempong E, Schwartz E (1980) Clinical features of thalassemia. Pediatr Clin North Am 27: 403
40. Leon MB, Borer JS, Bacharach SL, Green MV, Benz EJ, Griffith P, Nienhuis AW (1979) Detection of early cardiac dysfunction in patients with severe beta-thalassemia and chronic iron overload. N Engl J Med 301: 1143
41. Lewis BS, Rachmilewitz EA, Amitai N, Halon DA, Gotsman MS (1979) Left ventricular function in β-thalassemia and the effect of multiple transfusions. Am Heart J 96: 636
42. Lewis JR, Parker JO, Burggraf GW (1978) Mitral valve motion and changes in left ventricular end-diastolic pressure: a correlative study of the PR-AC interval. Am J Cardiol 42: 383
43. Lewis RP, Sandler H (1971) Relations between changes in left ventricular dimensions and the ejection fraction in man, Circulation 44: 548
44. Linhart JW, Mintz GS, Segal BL, et al. (1975) Left ventricular volume measurement by echocardiography: fact or fiction? Am J Cardiol 36: 114
45. McDonald RA, Mallory GK (1960) Hemochromatosis and hemosiderosis: study of 211 autopsied cases. Arch Intern Med 105: 686
46. Malamos B, Fessas P, Stamatoyannopoulos G (1962) Types of thalassemia trait carriers as revealed by their incidence in Greece. Br J Haematol 8: 5
47. Modell CB (1977) Total management of thalassemia. Arch Dis Child 52: 489
48. Propper RD, Button NL, Nathan DG (1980) New approaches to the transfusion management of thalassemia. Blood 55: 55
49. Richter GW (1978) The iron loaded cell – the cytopathology of iron storage. Am J Pathol 91: 361
50. Sanghvi LM, Sharma R, Misra SN (1957) Cardiovascular disturbances in chronic severe anemia. Circulation 15: 373
51. Schizas N, Tegos K, Voutsadakis A, Arabatzis G, Angelopoulou P, Chrysanthopoulos K, Athanasiadou A, Bathrellou S, Rombos J, Scarlos D, Davakis M (1977) The frequency and distribution of β-thalassemia and abnormal hemoglobins in Greece. A study of 15500 recruits. Hell Armed Forces Med Rev (Suppl 1) 11: 197
52. Shellhammer RF, Engle MA, Hagstrom JW (1967) Histochemical studies of the myocardium and conduction system in acquired iron-storage disease. Circulation 35: 631

53. Stamatoyannopoulos G, Fessas P (1964) Thalassemia, glucose 6-phosphate dehydrogenase deficiency, sickling and malarial endemicity in Greece. A study of five cases. Br Med J 1: 875
54. Valdes-Cruz LM, Reinecke C, Rutkowski M, Dudell GG, Goldberg SJ, Allen HD, Sahl DJ, Piomelli S (1982) Preclinical abnormal segmental cardiac manifestations of thalassemia major in children transfusion-chelation therapy: echographic alterations of left ventricular posterior wall contraction and relaxation patterns. Am Heart J 103: 505
55. Varat MA, Adolph RJ, Fowier NO (1972) Cardiovascular effect of anemia. Am Heart J 83: 415

12 Radiological Aspects of Marrow Heterotopia in Thalassemia

C. Papavasiliou

Introduction

Synonyms of "marrow heterotopia" (MH) are "extramedullary hemopoiesis" and "myeloid metaplasia." The purpose of this paper is to review the subject of MH in β-Thalassemia. Although MH is not a new entity to the pathologists, it is a comparatively recent one from the clinical, radiological, and therapeutic standpoint. Lately, computerized tomography (CT) has contributed to a more thorough investigation of MH [20]. In this paper, MH will be reviewed on the basis of existing reports and the author's experience, extending over 20 years. MH occurs in about 16% of patients with thalassemia major or intermedia.

Pathology

The term "marrow heterotopia" refers to foci of hemopoiesis situated in tissues other than the medullary cavity of the bones. Extramedullary hemopoiesis usually shows a nodular pattern: the nodules consist of normoblasts or their precursors, myeloblasts, and megakaryocytes (Fig. 1), or all three elements together. It is considered as a compensatory phenomenon, encountered in chronic anemias accompanied by bone marrow insufficiency. However, at autopsies, extramedullary marrow has been demonstrated without an anemia being associated [2]. It is also a physiological phenomenon in babies and infants [2]. Table 1 lists the diseases associated with extramedullary hemopoiesis. The most common ones are various forms of thalassemia, spherocytic anemias, and myelofibrosis. The sites in which MH has been commonly observed are listed in Table 2. Usually, MH is evident only by microscopical examination, but sometimes it causes macroscopically visible tumorlike masses. Such masses have been seen in the retroperitoneal space, pelvis, falx cerebi, presacral space, and maxillary antra, but most commonly they are situated inside the thoracic cage.

Several theories have been advanced to explain the origin and development of these masses. Lyall [13] suggested that they develop according to Cohnheim's theory of tumor growth, i.e., by islets of marrow-forming tissues separating during development and coming to rest in other tissues. These "rests" later undergo proliferative changes in response to increased functional demand. According to another theory, embolic or metastatic dissemination of bone marrow takes place through the intercostal veins to form the masses of heterotopic marrow [2]. These two theories presuppose a lack of connection between masses of heterotopic marrow and the adjacent bone [7, 2]. Others, however, claim a definite connection between the masses and the marrow of the adjacent bone, rib or vertebra [5, 11, 14]. They postulate that the masses arise from the marrow of the adjacent bone. Personal experience, based on radiological observations, favors the latter theory.

Thus, in some of the tomograms, soft-tissue masses are clearly visible around the expanded posterior parts of the ribs. Also, in several other cases, smaller masses are situated adjacent to and around the expanded anterior parts of the ribs. In some cases, the soft-tissue mass has the appearance of a halo

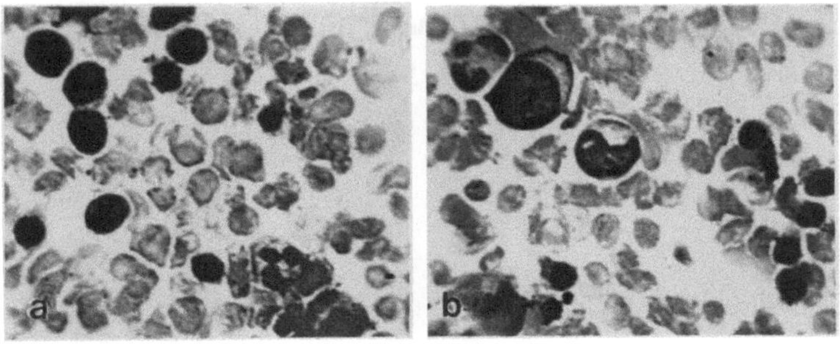

Fig. 1 a, b. Micrographs obtained by needle aspiration. Erythroblasts and leukoblasts of different maturation are seen

around either the anterior or posterior end of the rib. In thalassemia major, these parts of the ribs undergo the greatest expansion, as well as osteoporosis and trabeculation. The cortex becomes thinner and sometimes disappears altogether, and no clear-cut margin remains between the marrow masses and the rib. In one of our patients, CT showed that the anterior cortex of the rib at the site of the mass had disappeared, and flecks of bone were visible, displaced anteriorly (Fig. 6). It appears that the marrow "overflows" from the bone, destroys the cortex, and spreads around it, creating the masses. A similar process may start from a vertebral body. Radiological evidence favors a more consistent relationship between the rib and the masses: masses of heterotopic marrow have not been found adjacent to the cervical or lumbar vertebrae, and one is inclined to believe that it usually arises in the ribs rather than in the vertebral body.

It should be mentioned, however, that in two of our patients the cortex of the vertebra or rib adjacent to the masses was found intact. In addition, at autopsy, no connection was found between the masses and the adjacent bone in several cases [2]. Therefore, the theory that the masses of heterotopic marrow originate from metastatic marrow or from embryonal rests should not be disregarded. It is likely that both ways are at work: in most patients a direct spread takes place, while in others an embolic or "metastatic" process may be responsible. In addition, these two mechanisms may operate in the same patient.

Table 1. Diseases associated with extramedullary hemopoiesis [2]

Pernicious anemia during periods of relapse
Osteosclerosis
Myelophthisic anemia
Macrocytic anemia of hepatic origin
Carcinoma (with extensive bone marrow invasion)
Hodgkin's disease (with extensive bone marrow invasion)
Lymphoma (with extensive bone marrow invasion)
Leukemia (with extensive bone marrow invasion)
Osteitis cystica
Polycythemia
Erythroblastosis of the newborn
Spherocytic anemia
Myelofibrosis
Sickle cell anemia
Thalassemia etc.

Table 2. Sites of extramedullary hemopoiesis

Spleen
Liver
Lymph nodes
Hilum of kidneys
Thyroid
Minor pelvis
Pleura
Appendix
Retroperitoneal space
Falx cerebri
Costovertebral gutter
Anterior part of rib
Maxillary antra
Presacral space
Adrenals
Extradural space of spinal canal etc.

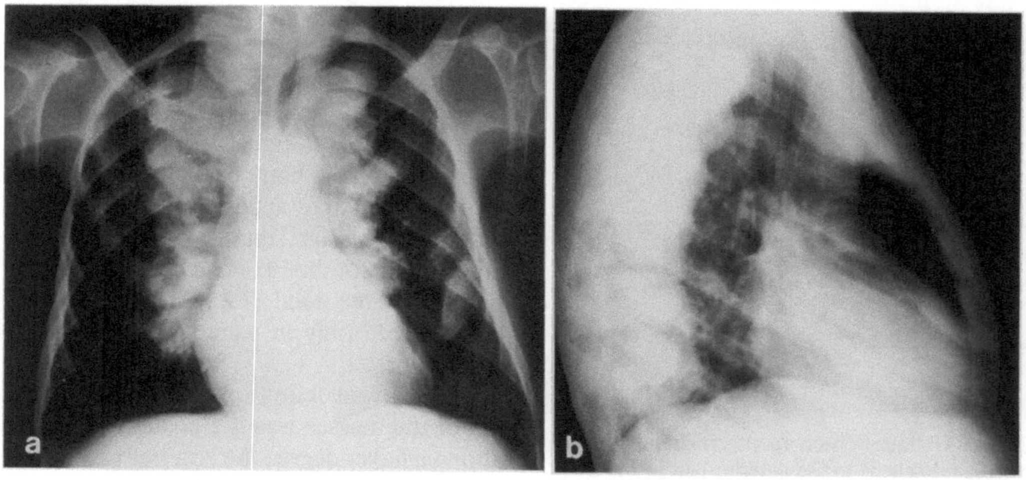

Fig. 2 a, b. Chest radiographs. Posteroanterior (**a**) an lateral view (**b**), showing multiple masses located in the costovertebral gutter bilaterally, presenting a segmental arrangement

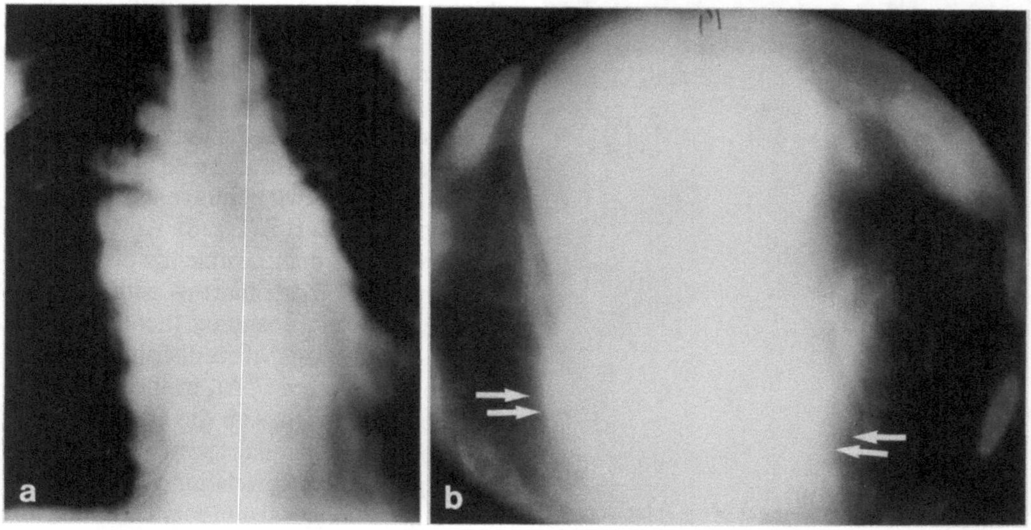

Fig. 3 a, b. Conventional laminograms. **a** Anteroposterior view, showing masses as a single density with lobulated borders located posteriorly. **b** Transverse view, showing masses in costovertebral angles (*arrows*)

Radiological Findings

Review of the literature and personal experience testifies that tumorlike masses of heterotopic bone marrow are situated in the posterior mediastinum, and particularly in the costovertebral angle. This was demonstrated in posteroanterior and lateral chest radiographs, in which the masses were located medially and posteriorly (Fig. 2). In laminograms, they appeared only in the posterior sections of the chest (Fig. 3). In transverse laminograms, the masses were clearly visualized in the costovertebral angles (Fig. 3). Most often they were multiple, having a soft-tissue density, with well-defined margins, and presenting a symmetrically segmental arrangement [16, 17]. In cases where superimposition occurred they appeared as a single density with lobulated borders (Fig. 3). In some cases, the masses lay

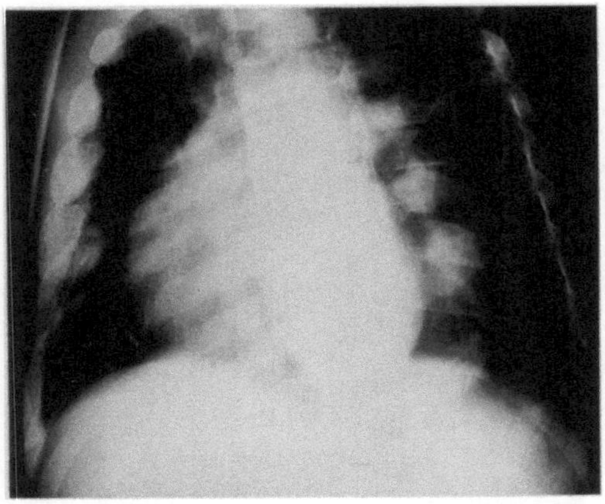

Fig. 4. Oblique chest roentgenogram, showing masses "attached" to the anterior part of the rib

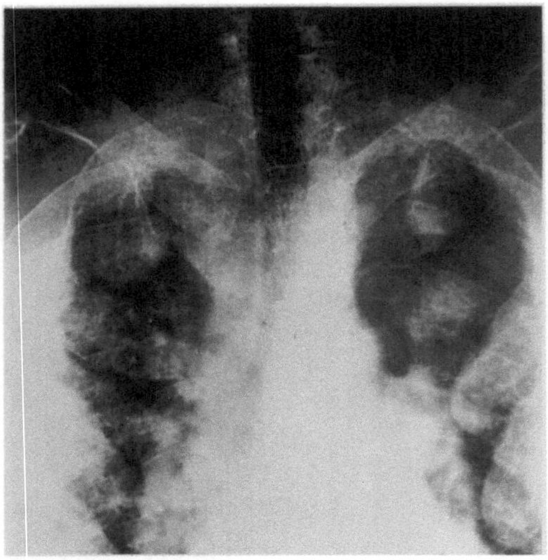

Fig. 5. Fingerlike appearance of the anterior part of the ribs

some cases, the masses lay consistently adjacent to the posterior part of the ribs. In several cases, smaller ovoid masses, 2–3 cm in diameter, were seen adjacent to the anterior part of several ribs (Fig. 4). This part and the corresponding posterior part of the rib undergo the greatest expansion and trabeculation in thalassemia major.

The most advanced cases were those which showed additional masses in the anterior part of the ribs. Another advanced case showed the mass as a halo around the expanded anterior part of the rib. In this case, the cortex of the anterior part of the rib was very indistinct due to osteoporosis and expansion. The masses of heterotopic marrow looked like "soft-tissue" prolongation and thickening of the bony part of the rib giving to it a "finger-like" appearance (Fig. 5). The latter findings, i.e., masses adjacent to the anterior part of the rib, have been previously noted and recorded [18]. They have been encountered only in patients with thalassemia major.

CT showed definite evidence that the origin of the masses was the posterior (Fig. 6) and to a lesser degree the anterior part of the rib. In one patient, using CT, we were able to demonstrate the presence of extramedullary hemopoiesis in the maxillary antra (Fig. 7). In this case, both antra were expanded and ballooned in a symmetrical manner. Conventional radiographs showed lack of pneumatization of these structures [1].

It is of interest that the mass in one of our patients was demonstrated on a thoracic scintiscan, made following intravenous injection of colloidal ^{198}Au [16] (Fig. 8). Kniseley at al. [9] were able to demonstrate the distribution of hemopoietic bone marrow with statisfactory detail by scintiscanning, thereby exploiting the observation that the distribution of intravenously injected ^{198}Au in the bone marrow correlated well with the areas of active hemopoiesis. A similar technique was used in our patient, and correlation was found between the radiological and scintiscanning findings. The appearance of the skull and pelvis of the same patient was typical of advanced thalassemia major. Currently, ^{59}Fe and ^{99m}Tc-labeled sulfur colloid are used for the investigation of marrow distribution in various pathological conditions [21].

The most commonly encountered CT findings were soft-tissue densities located in front of the posterior part of the ribs. The adjacent anterior cortex of the ribs, as already mentioned, was indistinct or completely destroyed (Fig. 6). In two of our patients, solitary or multiple masses were found in the costovertebral gutter, but there was no destruction of the adjacent cortex of the bone, vertebra or rib (Fig. 9). In another patient although some masses were associated with destruction of adjacent cortical rib bone, a separate mass was located adjacent to a vertebral body. In this latter location, there was no associated cortical bone destruction. According to our experience, masses which are not associated with destruction of adjacent bone are usually solitary and occur more often in thalassemia intermedia.

Comment

Tumor-simulating MH is an uncommon, although usually incidental, finding in chest radiographs of patients with thalassemia major. In a series of 98 thalassemic patients admitted to hospital, 18 possessed intrathoracic MH in the form of masses, an incidence of 16%. Radiological recognition of these masses of heterotopic marrow is imperative to rule out other masses, usually neoplastic, in the posterior mediastinum. Indeed, Knoblich [10] reported the case of a patient who underwent thoracotomy for a "neurogenic tumor of the posterior mediastinum." Histological examination of the excised mass showed the presence of heterotopic bone marrow, and the patient was found in retrospect to have thalassemia minor. If one is aware of the entity, the nature of the masses can easily by recognized, especially in association with the history of anemia, clinical picture, and other laboratory findings.

It should be mentioned that the bone findings (osteoporosis, trabeculation, etc.) in patients seen lately were less severe and occasionally quite inconspicuous. This has been attributed to the progress in the management of this disease in recent years. Tumors of the posterior mediastinum which should be differentiated from MH are listed in Table 3. In one of our patients, masses located at the anterior part of the rib had the appearance of bilateral "cannonball" lesions, and on the posteroanterior chest X-ray film they resembled pulmonary metastases (Fig. 10); however, lateral films showed that the masses were located anteriorly [18].

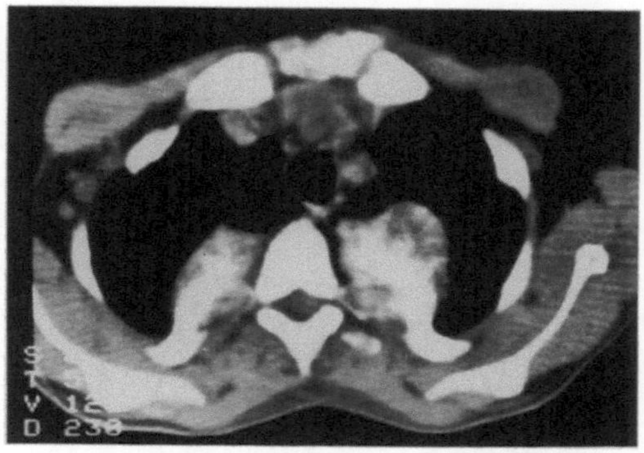

Fig. 6. CT. Soft-tissue mass of MH arising from the proximal part of the rib. Note destruction of the cortex of the rib

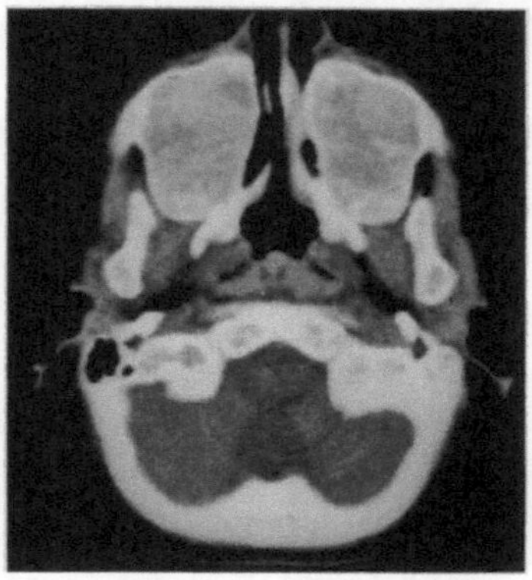

Fig. 7. MH masses in the maxillary antra. Note expansion of the bone walls

Table 3. Posterior mediastinal masses to be differentiated from MH [2]

Aneurysm
Neurogenic tumors
Tuberculous abscess
Carcinoma of bronchus
Extrapleural cysts
Endothelioma
Lipoma
Carcinoma of thyroid
Intrathoracic meningocele
Intrathoracic goiter
Myxochondroma
Myxochondrosarcoma
Benign lymph node hyperplasia

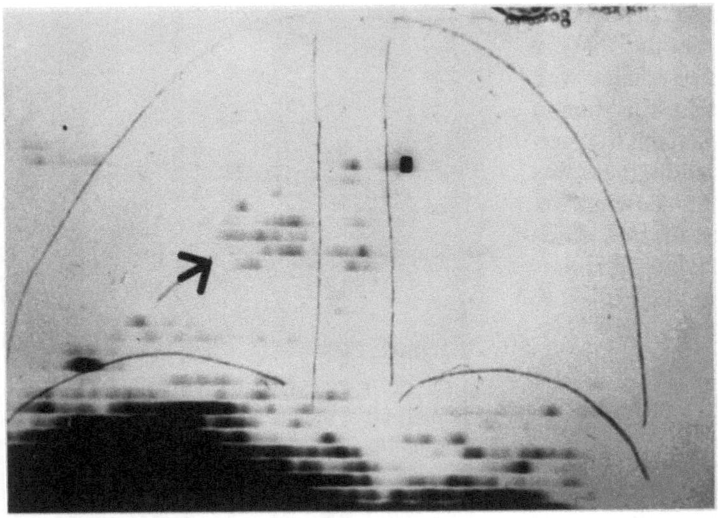

Fig. 8. Photoscan after injection of ^{198}Au revealing concentration of radioactive material in the mass of the right costovertebral gutter (*arrow*)

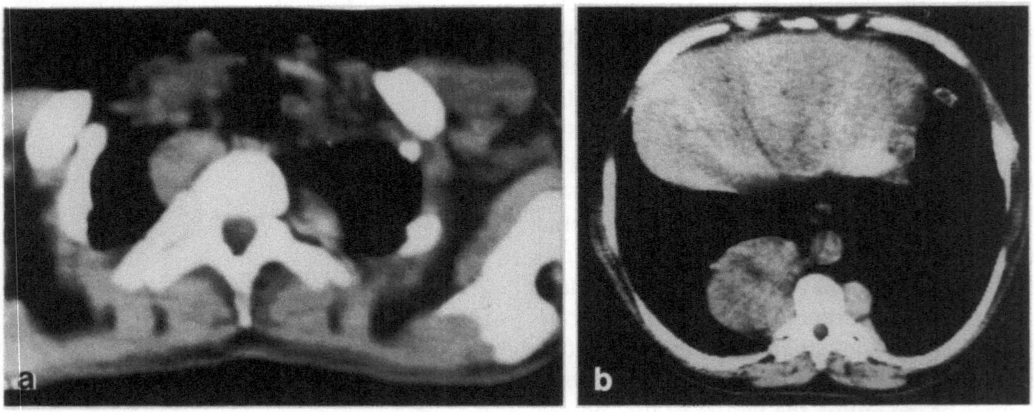

Fig. 9 a, b. Masses of MH adjacent to the vertebra. There is no erosion of the cortex of the bone

Although masses of heterotopic bone marrow are usually asymptomatic, in several patients they are associated with symptoms and signs of spinal cord compression of various degrees of clinical severity [4, 6, 8, 15, 22]. This is due to intrusion of MH into the spinal canal. A conventional or CT myelogram after intrathecal injection of metrizamide may reveal a block at the level of the thoracic spine (Fig. 11) or a constriction of the subarachnoid space (Fig. 12). Thoracic pain and even dyspnea caused by pressure of MH on the major airways have also been observed. Chao et al. [3] reported a case of MH located in the presacral area, causing constipation alternating with diarrhea. The treatment of choice for these complications of MH is radiotherapy in small doses [20].

In recent years, the outlook for thalassemia has improved considerably. The signs and symptoms of the disease are not so pronounced, and the survival time has increased. This is due to intense symptomatic treatment: patients have been receiving blood transfusion, and they undergo splenectomy and also removal of iron by desferrioxamine. Endocrinological and other metabolic disturbances are being corrected. Small doses of radiotherapy are able to relieve spinal cord compression, back pain and dyspnea due to masses of MH. We were struck by the fact that the expansion of the maxillary antra in

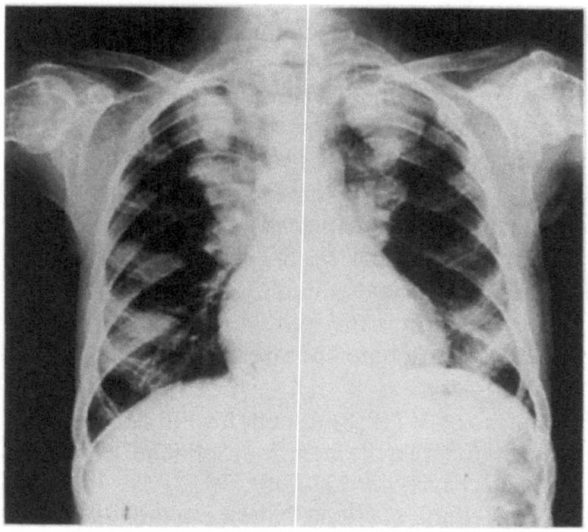

Fig. 10. Posteroanterior chest radiograph showing masses located at the anterior part of the ribs, quite separate from the mediastinum, resembling pulmonary metastases

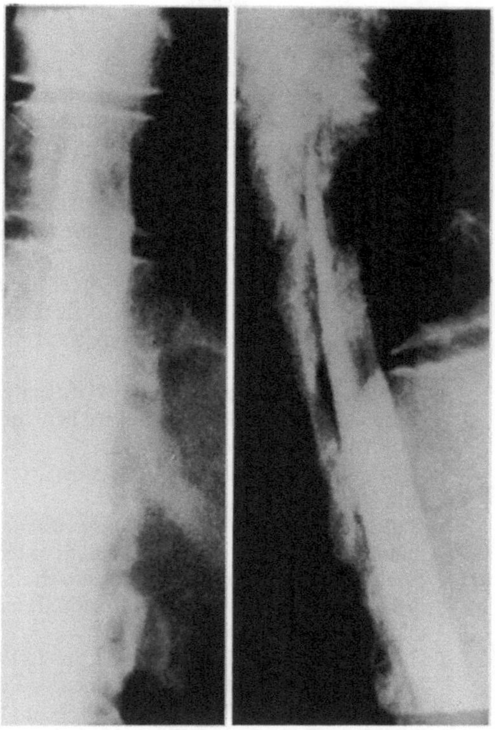

Fig. 11. Myelogram revealing obstruction at the level of T10 due to intrusion of MH into the spinal canal

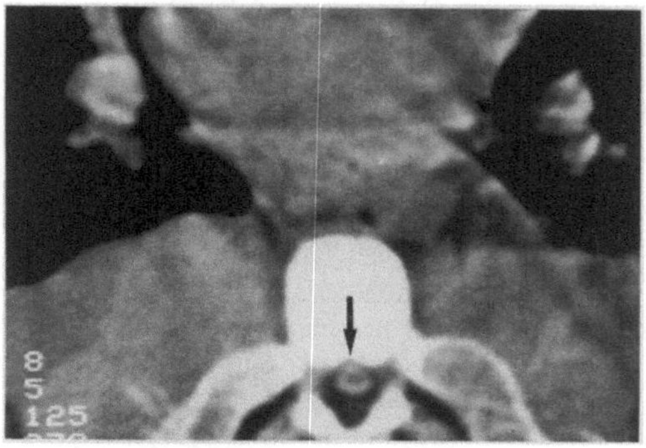

Fig. 12. Myelogram showing constriction of subarachnoid space due to mass of MH (*arrow*) in the extradural space

one of our patients was due to MH. One may speculate that some manifestations of the disease are due to compression by heterotopic marrow, e.g., pituitary dysfunction. If such is the case, radiotherapy in small doses could correct this abnormality as well.

Summary

The subject of MH has been reviewed on the basis of the author's experience and reports in the literature. Using conventional radiography, scintigraphy, CT, and myelography, 16% of the cases admitted to hospital with a diagnosis of thalassemia were found to have macroscopic masses of MH. The most common site of development of these masses was the costovertebral gutter, followed by the anterior end of the ribs and the extradural space of the spinal canal. The radiological findings, clinical implications, pathogenesis of the masses, and differential diagnosis from other tumorlike entities have been discussed.

References

1. Andreou J, Gouliamos A, Kalovidouris A, Papailiou J, Papavasiliou C (1984) Bone marrow hyperplasia of the maxillary sinuses in β-thalassemia. J Comput Assis Tomogr 8: 180
2. Ask-Upmark E (1945) Tumour simulating intrathoracic heterotopia of bone marrow. Acta Radiol (Stockh) 26: 425–440
3. Chao P, Farman J, Rapelner S (1986) CT features of presacral mass. An unknown focus of extramedullary hemopoiesis. J Comp Assist Tomogr 10: 684–687
4. Close A, Taira Y, Clevaland D (1958) Spinal cord compression due to extremedullary hematopoiesis. Ann Intern Med 48: 421–427
5. Fessas P, Loukopoulos D (1974) β-thalassemia. Clin Haematol 3: 411
6. Gatto J, Terrana V (1964) Compressione sil midollo spinale da proliferazione di midollo osseo nello spazio epidulare in sogetto affetto da malattia die Cooley splenectomizzatio. Haematologica (Pavia) 38: 61–75
7. Hanford R, Schneider G, MacCarthy J (1960) Massive thoracic extra-medullary hemopoiesis. N Engl J Med 263: 120–121
8. Irvin RA, Robertson WB (1964) Spinal cord compression in malignant lymphomas. Br Med J 1: 1354–1356
9. Kniseley RM, Andrews GA, Edwards CL, Tanida R (1964) Scanning of bone marrow hematopoietic disorders. IAEA Symposium on Medical Radioisotope Scanning, Athens
10. Knoblich R (1960) Extramedullary hemopoiesis presenting as intrathoracic mass. Report of case in patient with thalassemia minor. Cancer 13: 462–468
11. Litwer H (1969) Myelolipoma of the mediastinum. Radiology 74: 471–472
12. Lowman R, Bloor C, Newcomb A (1963) Roentgen manifestations of thoracic extramedullary hematopoiesis. Dis Chest 44: 154–162
13. Lyall A (1935) Massive extramedullary bonemarrow formation in a case of pernicious anemia. J Pathol Bacteriol 41: 469–470
14. Malmos B, Papavasiliou C, Avramidis A (1962) Tumour-simulating intrathoraic extramedullary hemopoiesis: report of case. Acta Radiol 57: 227–231
15. Marinozzi V (1958) Aspetti insoliti dell' iperplasia midollare nelle anemie emolitiche. Haematologica (Pavia) 43: 737–740
16. Papavasiliou C (1965) Tumour-simulating intrathoracic extramedullary hemopoiesis. AJR 93: 695–702
17. Papavasiliou C, Sfikakis P (1964) Tumour simulation intrathoracic marrow heterotopia in thalassemia major. Thorax 19: 121–124
18. Papavasiliou C, Konstantoulakis M, Priovolos J et al. (1979) The anterior costal margin mass in thalassemia major. Clin Radiol 30: 521–524
19. Papavasiliou C (1982) Radiotherapy of symptomatic tumor-simulating extramedullary hemopoiesis. Int J Radiat Oncol Biol Phys 8: 1813–1814
20. Papavasiliou C, Andreou J, Stringaris K, Vlahos L, Pontifex G (1982) The CT findings of extramedullary hematopoiesis. Radiologe 22: 86–87
21. Scutellari PN, Franceschini J, Orzincolo C (1982) Skeletal changes in treated β-thalassemia X-rays. Rome 13–25, 1982.
22. Sorsdahl OS, Taylor PE, Noyes WD (1964) Extramedullary hemopoiesis, mediastinal masses, spinal cord compression. J Am Med Assoc 189:343-347

13 Magnetic Resonance Imaging of Marrow Heterotopia in the Hemoglobinopathies

S. Trakadas, G. Pouliades, A. Gouliamos, L. Vlahos, J. Pappas, A. Aesopos, and C. Papavasiliou

Introduction

The radiological manifestations of tumor-simulating marrow heterotopia (MH) as seen on conventional radiography or computerized tomography (CT) have been described in detail in other parts of this chapter and by other investigators [4, 6, 8]. Magnetic resonance imaging (MRI) has great potential for clinical evaluation of bone marrow disorders. This is due to its inherently high contrast resolution, its lack of streak artifacts from thick cortical bone, and its proven utility in the evaluation of soft tissue neoplasms. Thus, three patients suffering from thalassemia major or sickle cell anemia and presenting MH were studied in our institution by MRI (Table 1).

Diagnostic Value of MRI

The MRI characteristics of marrow in adults approximate those of fat, that is, a short T_1 and relatively long T_2 [11]. Bone marrow in the healthy adult consists of a combination of hemopoietic and fatty marrow distributed in an age related pattern [5]. Since T_1 relaxation time of fat is slightly shorter than that of hemopoietic tissue, MRI may afford a unique opportunity to study bone marrow noninvasively [5]. The diffusely decreased signal of marrow in hemoglobinopathies is a reflection of hemopoietic marrow hyperplasia [2]. As primary marrow neoplasms, such as leukemia or lymphomas, increase marrow cellularity, areas of infiltration are satisfactorily manifested by decreased signals; therefore, MRI has been used in the study of these entities [11]. MRI has also been used in the study of both soft tissue neoplasms and mediastinal tumors [1, 12]. MRI displaying physiochemical properties unrelated to electron density may in the future distinguish benign from malignant solid mediastinal masses [2]. However, the present early MR intensity data and images do not show characteristics of either benignity or malignancy, and the T_1 and T_2 relaxation values and derived intensity data do not appear to be specific for individual pathological conditions [2]. The ability of MRI to obtain sagittal or coronal images directly is a unique advantage. It provides three-dimensional information on size and shape of lesions superior to that obtainable by multiplanar reconstruction of CT scans [10]. MRI, however, fails to depict soft tissue calcification and gas, and in this respect CT may yield additional information [2].

MH masses occur more commonly in thalassemia major or intermedia. In most instances, they are multiple and bilateral, originating from the posterior end of the rib [4, 6]. Radiologically (including CT), it is obvious that the hemopoietic tissue overflows the marow space, destroys the anterior cortex of the posterior part of the rib, and spreads ventrally to it [7]. Therefore, radiological pictures of the masses, in conjunction with osseous radiological findings and the clinical picture, are so characteristic that the diagnosis of MH is very apparent [7]. Occasionally, however, masses of MH may be solitary, not associated with the posterior part of the rib, and without cortical bone destruction. In addition, they may occur in patients with thalassemia minor [3]. In these cases, the diagnosis is not obvious, and a differential diagnosis from other posterior mediastinal masses should be

Table 1. Data for three patients with marrow heterotopia (MH)

	Patient		
	1	2	3
Type of anemia	Thalassemia major	Sickle cell anemia	Thalassemia intermedia
Age (years)/sex	34/M	27/F	24/M
Hemoglobin	9.4 g/liter	8.6 g/liter	10.1 g/liter
Conventional radiological findings[a]	Multiple thoracic paraspinal 4 to 5 cm masses	Multiple lower thoracic paraspinal 1 to 2 cm masses	Multiple lower thoracic paraspinal 1 to 2 cm masses
CT findings[a]	Masses originating from the posterior part of the ribs	Masses in the paraspinal region, some originating from the posterior part of ribs	CT not performed
Clinical symptoms[a]	None	Vague back pain	None

[a] Relevant to MH.

made. It was therefore thougt worthwhile to investigate the MRI appearance of MH. This information is of importance as radiotherapy may relieve symptoms of spinal cord compression or infiltration. Data reported in the literature do not provide the necessary information.

MRI Findings of MH

According to the experience in our institution, MRI appearance of MH is comparable to the findings observed on conventional radiography or on CT, i.e., delineation of bilateral, paraspinal, round, well-outlined masses, measuring from 1 to 5 cm in diameter. T_1-weighted images show low-intensity signal almost similar to that of the adjacent hypercellular marrow.

In sagittal planes, the masses project anteriorly. Most of these masses on T_1-weighted images were surrounded by a linear high-intensity signal, attributed to the presence of a layer of fat. As this high-intensity signal has not been observed in other benign or malignant tumors, or in space-occupying masses present in the mediastinum [1], it may be a characteristic sign of MH. However, this assumption should be substantiated by further observations. Although most masses were homogeneous, some of them presented foci of high-intensity signal, attributed again, to the presence of fat.

Figures 1–3 present MR images of three patients presenting MH without symptoms, suffering from thalassemia major, sickle cell anemia, and thalassemia intermedia respectively. There was good correlation between MR and conventional radiology or CT findings. As there was not clinical evidence of spinal cord infiltration in any of these patients, the question whether MRI can demonstrate spinal cord compression cannot be answered yet.

Summary

The MRI findings of MH masses are presented for three patients suffering from thalassemia major, sickle cell anemia, and thalasse-

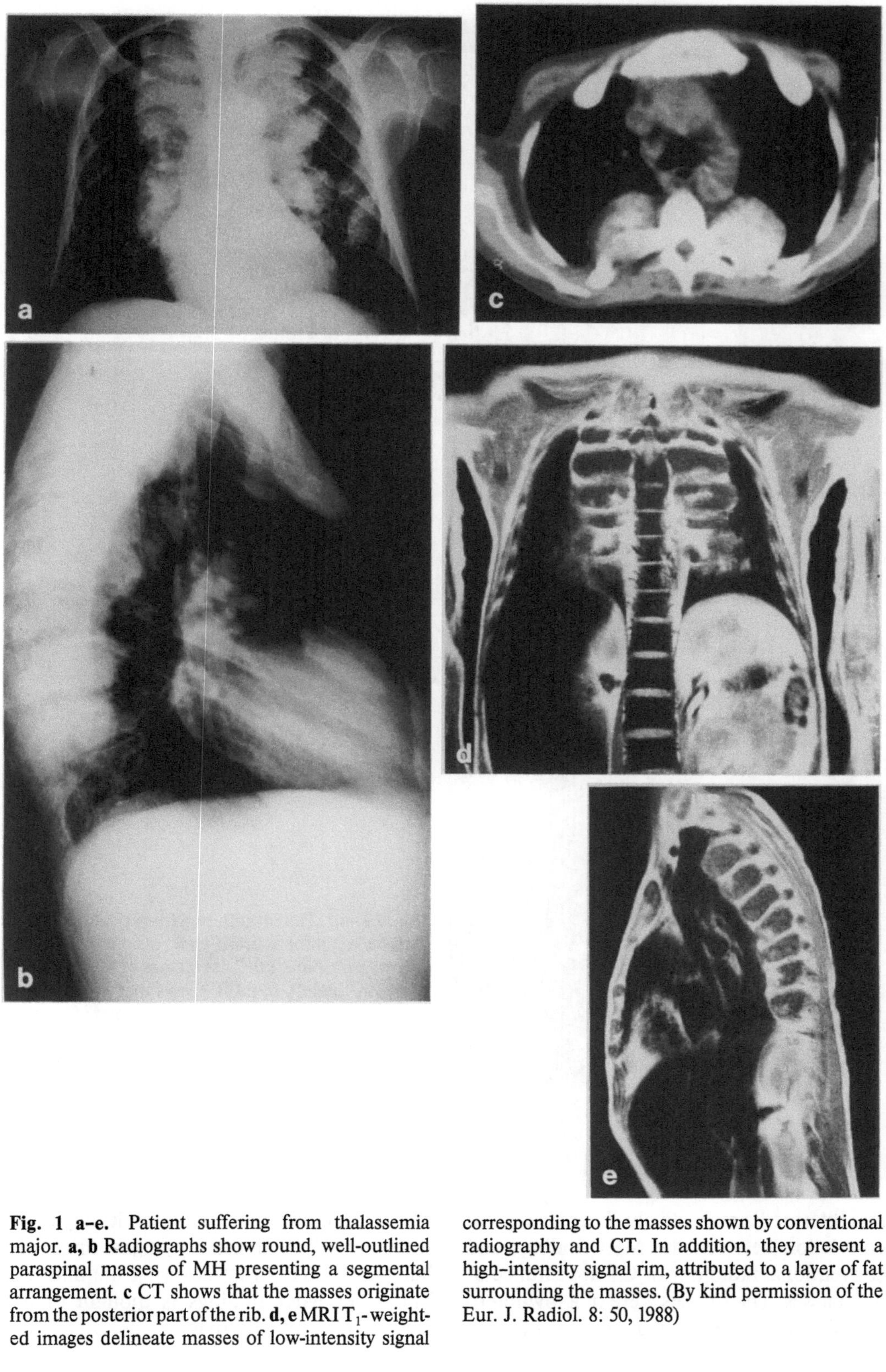

Fig. 1 a–e. Patient suffering from thalassemia major. **a, b** Radiographs show round, well-outlined paraspinal masses of MH presenting a segmental arrangement. **c** CT shows that the masses originate from the posterior part of the rib. **d, e** MRI T_1-weighted images delineate masses of low-intensity signal corresponding to the masses shown by conventional radiography and CT. In addition, they present a high-intensity signal rim, attributed to a layer of fat surrounding the masses. (By kind permission of the Eur. J. Radiol. 8: 50, 1988)

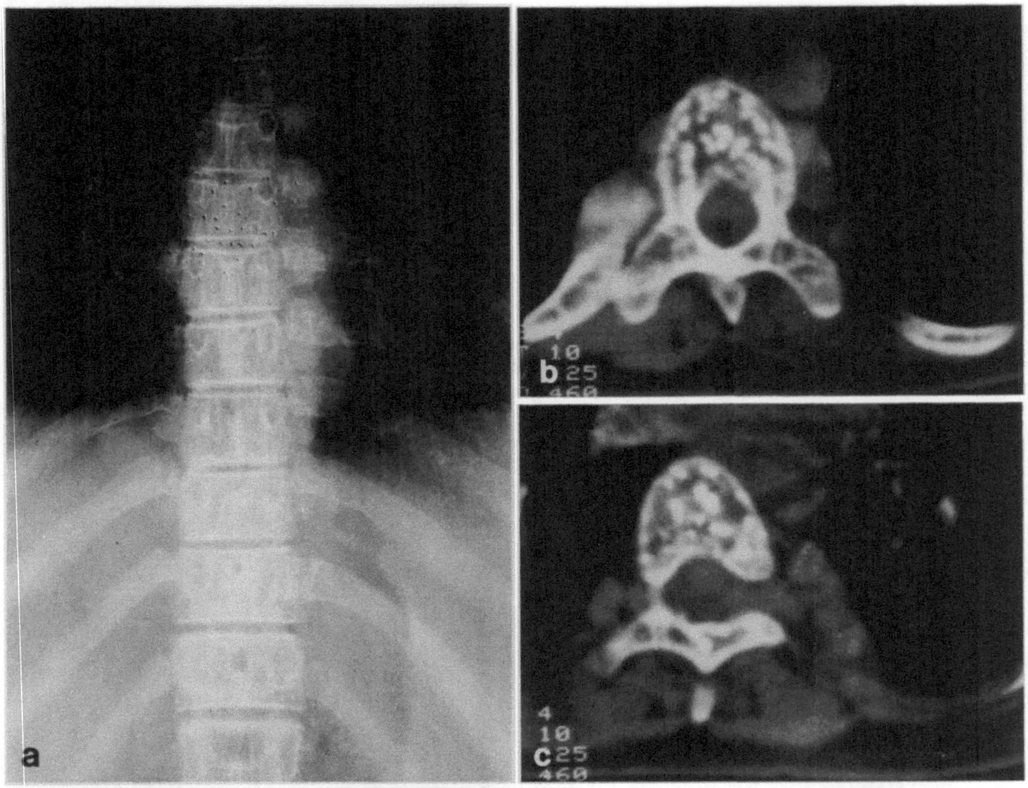

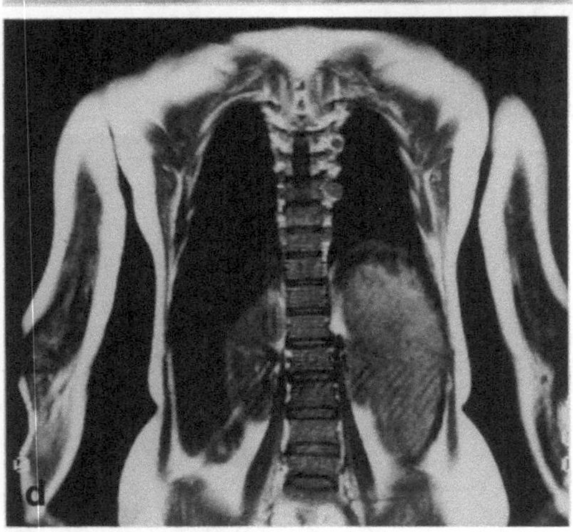

Fig. 2 a–d. Patient suffering from sickle cell anemia. **a** Anteroposterior view of thoracic spine shows paraspinal 1 to 2 cm masses of MH, particularly on the left. **b, c** CT shows that some of the massses originate from the posterior part of the rib. **d** MRI T_1-weighted image shows low-intensity signal masses surrounded by high-intensity signal rim

mia intermedia respectively. There was good correlation between the MRI findings and conventional radiology or CT appearance of the masses. The masses were of a low-intensity signal, similar to that of the adjacent marrow of the thoracic spine, while they were surrounded by high-intensity signal rim, attributed to a layer of fat covering the masses. The latter MRI findings is thought to be characteristic of MH masses.

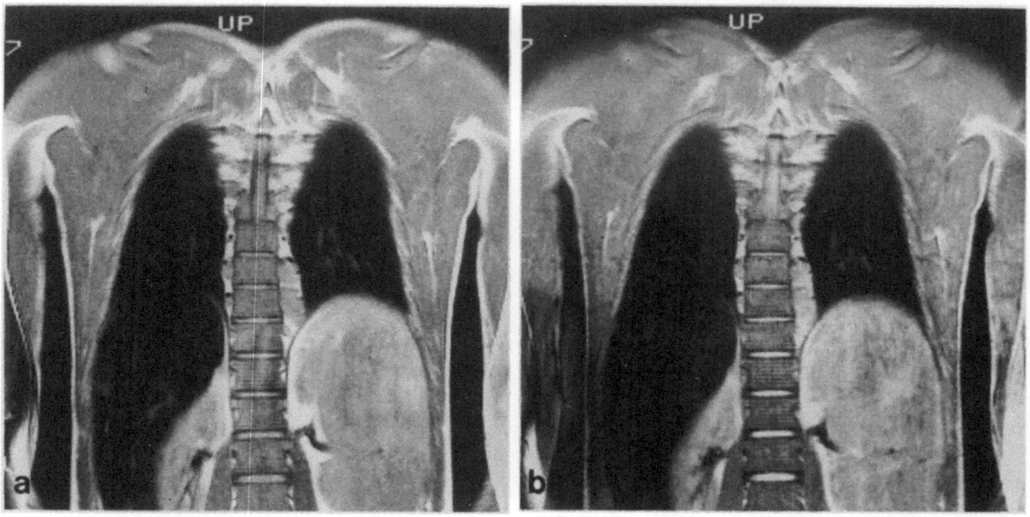

Fig. 3 a,b Patient suffering from thalassemia intermedia **a** MRI T_1- and **b** T_2-weighted images reveal 1 to 2 cm paraspinal masses of MH. The high-intensity signal rim is vaguely seen on T_1, and it is rather subtle on T_2. (By kind permission of the Eur. J. Radiol. 8: 50, 1988)

References

1. Gamsu G, Stark D, Webb WR, Moore EH, Sheldon P (1984) Magnetic resonance imaging of benign mediastinal masses. Radiology 151: 709-717
2. Kangarloo H, Dietrick R, Taira R, Gold RH, Lenarsky C, Boechat MI, Feig SA, Sulusky I (1986) MR imaging of bone marrow in children. J Comput Assist Tomogr 10: 205-209
3. Knoblich R (1960) Extramedullary hemopoeisis presenting as intrathoracic mass. Report of a case in patient with thalassemia minor. Cancer 13: 462-468
4. Lowman R, Bloor C, Newcomb A (1963) Roentgen manifestation of intrathoracic extramedullary hematopoiesis. Dis Chest 44: 154-162
5. Mitchell DF, Rao VW, Dalinka M, Spritner C, Axel L, Gefter W, Kricum M, Steinberg ME, Kressel HY (1986) Hematopoietic and fatty marrow distribution in the normal and ischemic hip. New observations with 1,5 T MR imaging. Radiology 161: 199-202
6. Papavasiliou CG (1965) Tumor-simulating intrathoracic extrmedulary hemopoiesis. A J R 93: 227-231
7. Papavasiliou C, Gouliamos A, Andreou J (1968) The marrow heterotopia in thalassemia. Eur J Radiol 6: 92-96
8. Papavasiliou C, Sandilos P (1987) Effect of radiotherapy on symptoms due to heterotopic marrow in β-thalassmia. Lancet I: 13-14
9. Papavasiliou C, Andreou J, Stringaris K, Vlahos L, Pontifex G (1982) The CT Findings of extramedullary hemopoieses. Radiologe 22: 86-87
10. Patasnick JR, Turner D, Charter J, Gitelis S, Zacharias CE (1986) Soft tissue masses of the locomotor system, comparison of MR imaging with CT. Radiology 160: 125-133
11. Porter B, Shields A, Olson D (1986) Magnetic resonance imaging of bone marrow disorders. Radiol Clin North Am 24: 269-289
12. Totty W, Murphy E, Lee J (1986) Soft tissue tumors. MR imaging.Radiology 160: 135-141

Part III

Management and Prevention

14 Effect of Radiotherapy on Symptoms due to Marrow Heterotopia in β-Thalassemia

C. Papavasiliou

Introduction

Extramedullary hemopoiesis or marrow heterotopia (MH) occurs in about 15% of cases of thalassemia major or intermedia [6, 8, 9]. It also occurs in myelosclerosis and in other chronic anemic conditions [2]. MH occurs usually in microscopic forms but occasionally in macroscopic tumor like masses located in various tissues and organs, more commonly in the thorax. Although MH is usually asymptomatic for long periods, it sometimes presents symptoms and signs of pressure on adjacent healthy tissue, particularly on the spinal cord. If present, this clinical expression depends on the location and size of the overgrowth. As hemopoietic tissue is sensitive to irradiation, radiotherapy has been used to relieve these symptoms [3–5, 6, 8, 10, 12].

Spinal Cord Compression

Several cases of spinal cord compression (SCC) due to MH have been reported. The usual location of the block is the thoracic spinal cord, particularly its lower part. Patients present with motor and sensory disturbances in the lower extremities, difficulty in walking, with urination, etc. Neurological examination discloses various degrees of muscular atrophy, weakness of both legs, and sensory loss below the spinal cord blockade. It may also reveal abnormal deep tendon reflexes and other pyramidal tract signs. In extreme cases there may be complete paraplegia of the lower extremities. There is usually good correlation between the level of spinal cord blockade and the location of the masses of MH as seen on chest or spinal radiographs. However, cases of SCC have been reported that were not associated with radiographic evidence of masses.

The exact location of the spinal cord block can usually be determined by conventional myelography or myelography using computerized tomography (CT) scan. CT myelography shows constriction of the subarachnoid space due to pressure by the masses located at the extradural space. The heterotopic tissue apparently originates from the masses located at the costovertebral gutter or the posterior end of the ribs which impinge into the spinal canal. Nuclear magnetic resonance imaging (MRI) may potentially delineate such masses more satisfactorily than conventional or CT radiography. The transverse myelitis encountered in thalassemia should be differentiated from the Guillain-Barré syndrome or transverse myelitis with spontaneous recovery. The clinical picture and relevant laboratory investigation will help in differential diagnosis. Compression due to collapse of a vertebra caused by osteopenia should also be ruled out.

Mild cases of SCC can be relieved by blood transfusions. Blood transfusion causes suppression of erythropoietin production, which leads to regression of the size of the masses and relief of the symptoms. However, improvement after blood transfusions may be slow or is incomplete, and the symptoms may recur if the transfusion regimen is suspended. Surgical removal and decompression have been performed, usually before the exact diagnosis was made. Recovery after surgery is incomplete. This has been attributed to the

Table 1. Data for eight patients given radiotherapy for symptoms of MH (ref. 11)

Patient no.	Age (years)	Sex	Radiotherapy	TDF	Symptoms and results
1	14	F	9 Gy in 9 sessions in 11 days	10	SCC. Relief of Symptoms for 4 years
2	28	M	10.05 Gy in 11 sessions in 13 days	8.5	SCC. Relief of symptoms FU for 3 years
3	22	M	10 Gy in 7 sessions in 9 days	13	SCC. Relief of symptoms for 3 months
			15.5 Gy in 10 sessions in in 12 days	22	New course of radiotherapy after recurrence. Relief of symptoms. FU for 10 months
4	28	M	12 Gy in 6 sessions in 8 days and 4 Gy in SS 1 month later	24	SCC. Relief of symptoms for 1 year
5	50	M	6 Gy in SS, 6 Gy in SS 1 week later, and 6 Gy in SS 1 month later	30.5	SCC. Relief of symptoms for 1 year
6	59	M	14 Gy in 7 sessions in 9 days, 6 Gy in SS 1 month later, and 6 Gy in SS 2 months later	37	Dyspnea. Relief of symptoms for 9 months
7	49	M	10 Gy in 10 sessions in 12 days	11	Back pain. Relief of symptoms for 6 months
8	41	M	10 Gy in 10 sessions in 12 days	11	Back pain. Relief of symptoms for 6 months

FU, Follow-up; TDF, time-dose fractionation (based on the Nominal Standard Dose formula); SS, single session

diffuse nature of the process, which does not allow radical removal of MH. For the same reason, a recurrence of symptoms may take place soon after treatment. Sorsdahl [13] suggests, therefore, that irradiation should also be applied shortly after surgical decompression. As we have treated our patients with radiotherapy alone, we report two typical cases, taken from those listed in Table 1.

Patient No. 4

A 28-year-old male who had been suffering from thalassemia major since childhood was treated regularly with blood transfusions and desferrioxamine. For 6 months, he complained of some difficulty in walking and numbness of the lower extremities. Sensory disturbances were found at the level of T10 and below. There was a positive Babinski sign, particularly on the right side, and ankle clonus. A more detailed neurological examination established the diagnosis of a mild but definite SCC syndrome at the level of the T10 vertebra. Radiographs of the chest and thoracic spine revealed a mass, most likely MH, located adjacent to the T9–T10 vertebrae on the left side, and another mass in the right upper mediastinun, adjacent to the upper thoracic vertebrae. Hematocrit (Hct) was 36%, and WBC was 12×10^9/liter. The other clinical and laboratory findings were compatible with the patient's long-standing anemia. It was decided to treat the lower thoracic spine with irradiation. Using the cesium unit, 12 Gy were given by a posterior field in six sessions in 8 days. Although the patient became asymptomatic and there was definite improvement of his neurological symptomatology, radiographs revealed 1 month later that the mass of MH was still present, probably a little smaller. For this reason, 4 Gy were given in one session. Radiographs revealed complete disappearance of the mass (6 months later) The patient continued to be asymptomatic (Fig. 1 a–c).

Patient No.5

A 50-year-old male was diagnosed as having suffered from thalassemia major since the age of 6 years. He had recently been complaining of motor disturbances and numbness of the lower extremities, particularly the right leg. Some muscular atrophy was present. There was no Babinski sign. A posteroanterior radiograph of the chest revealed a large mass – presumably MH – located in the right lower posterior mediastinum paraspinally. CT revealed a 5 x 8 cm mass, located at the level of T8–T10 vertebrae. CT after intrathecal injection of metrizamide revealed constriction of the subarachnoid space, at the same level, apparently by masses of MH intruding into the spinal canal from the costovertebral gutter. Radioisotopic liver scan revealed enlargement of the liver, particularly the left lobe, and also irregular uptake. Other clinical and laboratory findings were consistent with the patient's chronic anemia: Hct was 31%, while WBC was 36, 5×10^9/liter.

The neurological symptoms were attributed to pressure from the mass located in the lower thoracic spine, and it was decided to treat the patient with irradiation. Using the cesium unit, 6 Gy were given in one session, and 1 week later the same dose was repeated, also in one session. The mass was still present and was relatively unchanged 1 month later; therefore, 6 Gy were given in one session. After 3 months, there was no more radiological evidence of the mass (Fig. 2 a–d), and the neurological symptoms and signs had regressed. The patient continued to be asymptomatic 1 year after radiotherapy (Fig. 2e).

In our opinion, radiotherapy is the treatment of choice for SCC. The good results obtained with this method are due to the radiosensitivity of bone marrow. When the entire bone marrow is exposed to irradiation, the lethal dose (LD) in 50% of patients in 30 days is 10 Gy [12]; however, with segmental irradiation, the dose required to make the marrow permanently aplastic is not known. Although even 1 Gy is sufficient to arrest mitosis, regeneration may take place even after exposure to 40–45 Gy [12].

Ectopic marrow may be more vulnerable than bone marrow [7]. Radiosensitivity may also vary according to location [8]. Rubin and Scarantino [12] reported that regeneration of the marrow after irradiation is the result of heterotypical conversion of mesenchymal cells in the local haversian canals and endosteum to stem cells.

Issargarisil et al. [5] treated 12 patients who suffered from SCC mostly with irradiation. The dose given ranged between 15 and 35 Gy and resulted in relief of symptoms in all patients. However, in some patients there was recurrence of symptoms, which necessitated a new course of radiotherapy. These authors do not provide any radiotherapeutic details. Two of their patients underwent surgical decompression and postoperative irradiation, while other patients were treated with blood transfusions. The authors concluded that the treatment of choice for SCC due to MH is radiation therapy alone, not preceded by surgery. They recommend a dose ranging from 20 to 30 Gy. The treatment field should cover

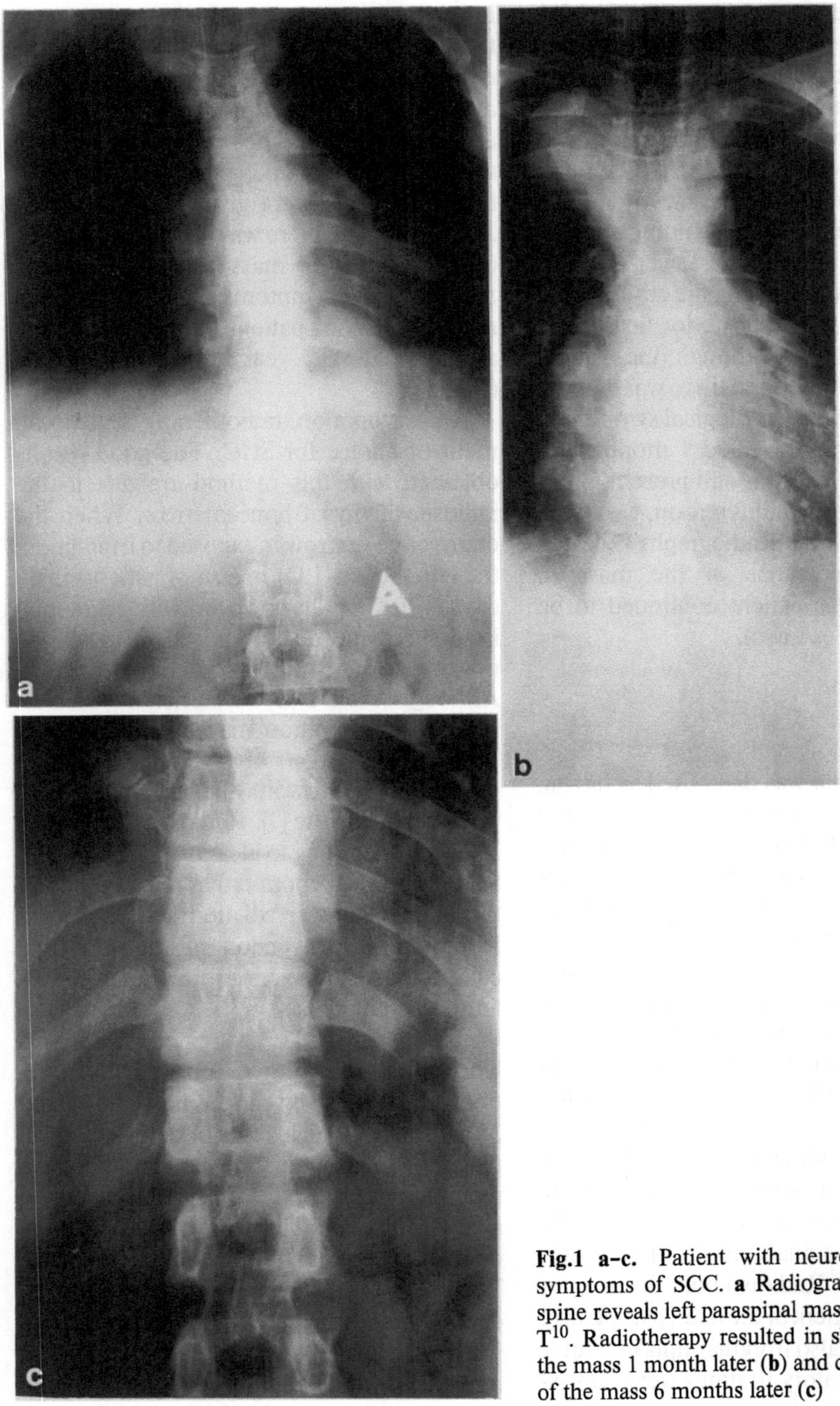

Fig.1 a–c. Patient with neurological signs and symptoms of SCC. **a** Radiograph of the thoracic spine reveals left paraspinal mass at the level of T^9–T^{10}. Radiotherapy resulted in slight diminution of the mass 1 month later (**b**) and complete resolution of the mass 6 months later (**c**)

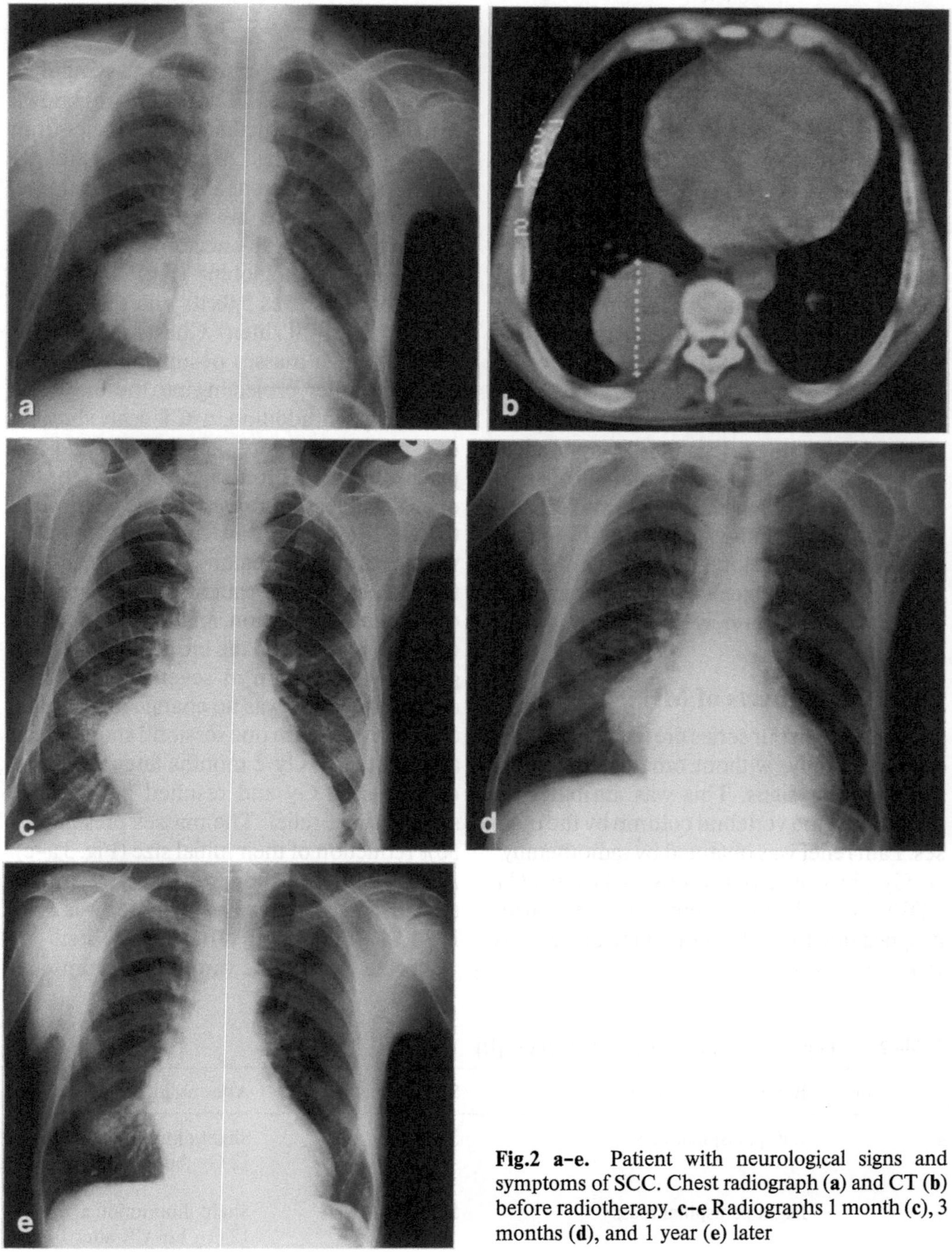

Fig.2 a–e. Patient with neurological signs and symptoms of SCC. Chest radiograph (**a**) and CT (**b**) before radiotherapy. **c–e** Radiographs 1 month (**c**), 3 months (**d**), and 1 year (**e**) later

the upper level of the spinal cord block as indicated by neurological examination and the lower level as demonstrated by myelography.

Papavasiliou and Sandilos [11] used doses ranging from 10 to 36 Gy (8,5–37 time-dose fractionation (TDF). There was prompt relief of symptoms in all patients except one, in whom a recurrence of symptoms was observed after 3 months, and who was treated again successfully with irradiation. The diagnosis in three of the total of five patients treated was established by CT-guided fine-needle biopsy. In the other two patients, the clinical and radiological findings were also so typical of MH that cytological diagnosis was not deemed necessary. There was good correlation between the radiological findings and estimation of the level of the block by neurological examination; therefore, only two of the five patients were subjected to myelography. Four patients however, were subjected to CT.

Other Side Effects of MH

Two patients in our series presented with thoracic pain only, without other neurological symptoms or signs. This was attributed to pressure on the vertebral column by the masses. Pain relief was obtained by radiotherapy; 10 Gy given in ten sessions in 12 days (11 TDF). One of our patients presented with dyspnea due to obstruction of the airways, as reported below.

Patient No.6

A 59-year old male presented with symptoms of respiratory distress. The patient was known to have suffered from thalassemia major from an early age and had been treated regularly with blood transfusions and desferrioxamine. Six months before his last admission, the patient underwent splenectomy. Ht was 35%, while the hemoglobin (Hb) level was 11 g/liter. RBC was $5{,}0 \times 10^{12}$/liter and WBC was $15{,}3 \times 10^{9}$/liter. Chest radiographs revealed huge masses occupying the costovertebral gutter, projecting into the lung fields bilaterally. In addition, a CT scan showed, that the masses were compressing and displacing the main bronchi, particularly the left one. No atelectasis or obstructive pneumonitis was present. On auscultation, a wheeze was heard over the region of the bifurcation of the trachea. As the patient was complaining of dyspnea on exertion, and this was attributed to the pressure on the bronchi, 14 Gy were given by irradiation in seven sessions in 9 days. Since there was no change in the mass, 6 Gy were given in one session 1 month later, and another 6 Gy 2 months later. The total dose was 26 Gy and resulted in complete symptomatic relief. The masses presented a 50% reduction of their initial size (Fig. 3 a–e). A blood examination performed 1 month after irradiation revealed that Hct was 35%, Hb 13.1 gr/liter, and WBC 30×10^{9}/liter.

Table 1 shows the various symptoms and

Table 2. Radiographic changes after radiotherapy [11]

Patient no.	Before radiotherapy	Size of masses	After radiotherapy
4	Left paraspinal mass	3 x 6 cm	Slight diminution after 12 Gy, but CR after 16 Gy
5	Right paraspinal mass	5 x 8 cm	Slight diminution after 12 Gy, but CR after 18 Gy
6	Huge paraspinal mass	15 x 22 cm	Unchanged after 14 Gy, slight diminution after 20 Gy, and almost 50% regression after 26 Gy

CR, Complete resolution

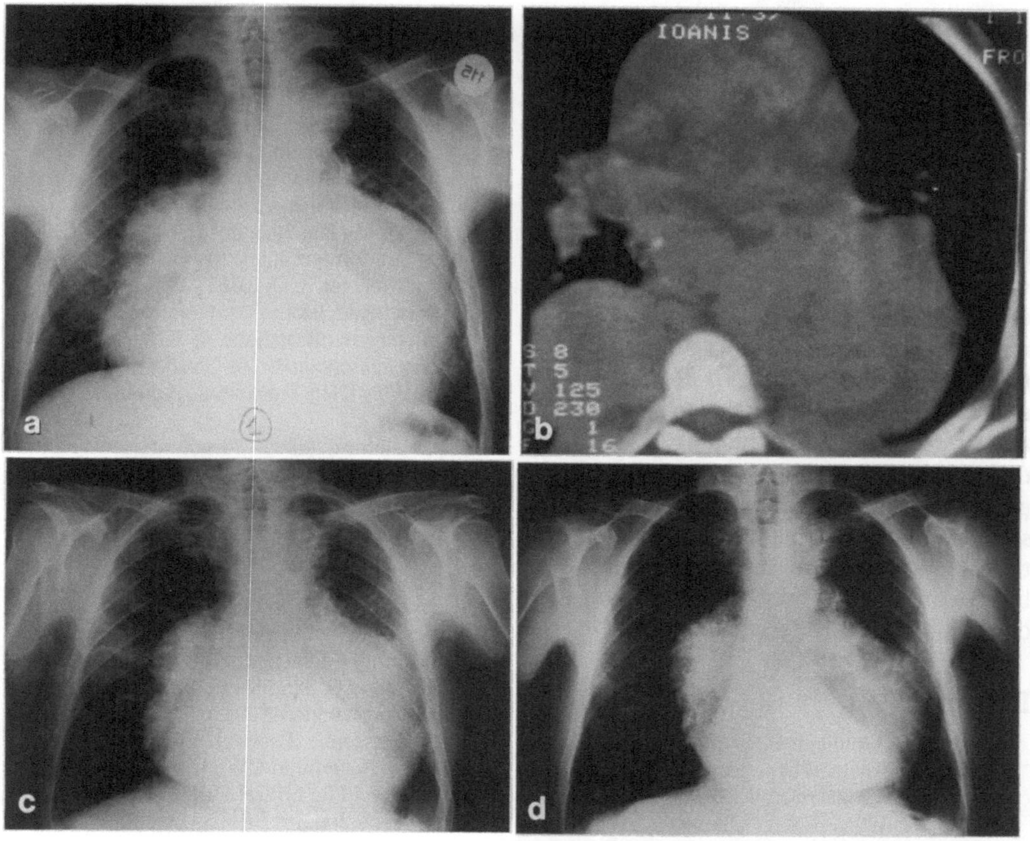

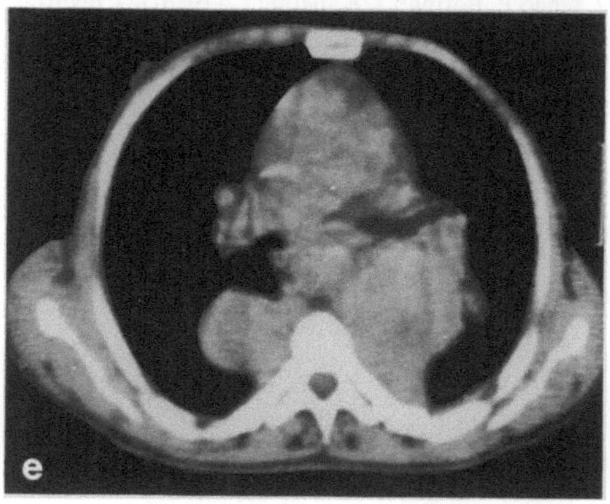

Fig.3 a–e. Patient presenting with dyspnea. Chest radiograph (**a**) and CT (**b**) reveal huge paraspinal masses invading the mediastinum and the lung. Radiotherapy resulted in slight diminution of the masses after 2 months (**c**) and almost 50% regression after 6 months (**d, e**).

the doses and results of radiotherapy in a group of eight patients treated in our institution. The size of the masses in three of the eight patients has been followed up by serial radiography. The results are seen in Table 2. In two patients there was complete, and in one patient a partial regression. Another reported complication attributed to MH is constipation due to pressure on the rectum by masses located in the presacral space (2). One of our patients, who presented with vague symptoms of nasal discomfort, was found to have masses of MH located in the maxillary antra [1].

Summary

Although patients with MH are usually asymptomatic, they may sometimes present with symptoms and signs of pressure on organs, mainly the spinal cord. Small doses of radiation may relieve the symptoms and restore neurological function. Radiotherapy may also relieve back pain due to pressure on the vertebral column by the masses, dyspnea due to obstruction of the major airways, and potentially other symptoms. Radiotherapy should be given with caution, and its effect on the blood should be monitored since the heterotopic marrow may be an important site of hemopoiesis for these patients.

References

1. Andreou J, Gouliamos A, Kalovidouris A et al. (1984) Bone marrow hyperplasia of the maxillary sinuses in *β*-thalassemia. J Comput Assist Tomogr 8: 180
2. Chao P, Forman J, Kapelner C (1986) CT features of the presacral mass. An unknown focus of extramedulary hemopoiesis. J Comput Assist Tomogr 10: 684–685
3. Close AS, Taira Y, Cleveland DA (1958) Spinal cord compression due to extramedullary hemopoiesis. Ann Intern Med 18: 421–427
4. Gatto J, Terrana V, Biondi L (1964) Compressione sul midollo spinal da proliferazione di midolloosseo spacio epidulare in soggeto affeto di maladia a Cooley splenoctomizatto. Haematologia (Pavia) 38: 61–75
5. Issargarisil S, Piankijagum A, Wasi P (1981) Spinal cord compression in thalassemia. Arch Intern Med 14: 1033–1036
6. Lowman RM, Bloor CM, Newcomb AN (1963) Roentgen manifestations of thoracic extramedullary hemopoiesis. Dis Chest 44: 154
7. Moss WT (1959) Therapeutic radiology. Mosby, St. Louis
8. Papavasiliou C (1965) Tumor simulating extramedullary hemopiesis. AJR 93: 695–702
9. Papavasiliou C, Konstantoulakis M, Priovolos J et al. (1979) The anterior costal margin mass in patients with thalassemia major. Clin Radiol 30: 521–524
10. Papavasiliou C (1982) Radiotherapy of symptomatic tumor simulating extramedullary hemopoiesis. Int J Radiat Oncol Biol Phys 8: 1813–1814
11. Papavasiliou C, Sandilos P (1987) Effect of radiotherapy on symptoms due to heterotopic marrow in *β*-thalassemia. Lancet I: 13–14
12. Rubin P, Scarantino CW (1978) The bone marrow organ. The critical structure in radiation-drug interaction. Int J Radial Oncol Biol Phys 4: 3–23
13. Sordahl OS, Taylor PE, Moyes WD (1964) Extramedullary hemopoiesis, mediastinal masses and spinal cord compression. JAMA 189: 343–347

15 Bone Marrow Transplantation for Thalassemia Major: The Place of Irradiation

Y. Rombos

Introduction

Standard treatment of thalassemia involves frequent blood transfusions to correct anemia and suppress marrow hyperactivity. Chronic iron chelation reduces or prevents hemosiderosis caused by this form of therapy. With this conventional treatment, life expectancy may exceed more than 25 years, and many patients manage to maintain normal activity and, occasionally, to raise families.

Since the thalassemic lesion is expressed only in the erythropoietic cell and all morbid manifestations derive directly or indirectly from this very specific defect, the idea of effecting a cure through cell replacement, i.e., bone marrow transplantation (BMT), has been entertained over the last 10–15 years.

In 1982, Thomas et al. [1] reported the first successful BMT for thalassemia major in a 16-month-old, minimally transfused Italian male. This success has led other groups to treat patients by high-dose chemotherapy or chemoradiotherapy followed by transfusion of hemopoietic stem cells, usually collected from human leukocyte antigen (HLA)-identical siblings of the affected child. Some of the results will be reviewed in this paper. In addition, future directions for the use of BMT in thalassemia major will be briefly discussed, including the place of preparative irradiation.

General Principles

Selection of Donors and Recipients

Thomas et al. [1] postulated that transplantation early in the course of the disease would result with a high probability in disease-free survival. In 1983, Lucarelli et al. [2] appeared to obtain no long-term survivors among thalassemic patients receiving transplants at a relatively advanced age. In this case, preparative regimens included total body irradiation (TBI). Recently, however, Lucarelli et al. [3, 4] were able to show that long-term disease-free survival may be possible in a high percentage of patients with advanced thalassemia major who receive transplants from HLA-matched siblings after preparation with busulfan (BU) and cyclophosphamide (CY) only.

More recently, in view of the fact that only 28% of patients have a histocompatible donor (HLA-identical sibling), transplants are being attempted using as donors family members who genotypically share only one HLA haplotype with the recipient and display phenotypic identity for one or two but not all of the other HLA determinants. Also, a few transplants have been carried out using unrelated donors who are phenotypically identical for HLA-A, -B, -C, or -D and -DR. Another possibility is to use a partially HLA-matched donor, as demonstrated by the Seattle group. These patients apparently have the same risk of graft-versus-host disease (GVHD) and of rejection as the perfectly matched ones [5]. Thus, the probability of finding suitable donor increases to about 40%.

Conditioning Regimens for Marrow Grafting

In patients with thalassemia, the aim would be to destroy genetically abnormal marrow and replace it with normal marrow from another individual. For marrow grafting to be

Table 1. Conditioning regimens used in preparation for BMT

Reference	No. of patients	Age	Regimen
Thomas et al. (1, 13)	5	13 months - ?	BU + CY, MTX
Lucarelli et al. (7)	30	6 months - 8 years	BU + CY, MTX or MTX + CY
Lucarelli et al. (4)	57 35 22	6 months - 8 years 8 months - 14 years	BU + CY, MTX or MTX + CY, OSA
Lucarelli et al. (3)	40	8–15 years	BU + CY, MTX, CY, CSA
di Girolamo et al. (11)	15	1–7 years	BU + CY, CSA
Slavin and Rachmilewitz (6)	4	9 months - 13 years	BU + TLI* + CY, depletion of T-lymphocytes
Lin et al. (10)	10	19 months - 13 years	BU + CY + TBI**, CSA, MTX, BU + CY

* TLI, total lymphoid irradiation, ** TBI, total body irradiation, 1 Patient

successful, sufficient immunosuppression must be provided. The conditioning regimens used for this purpose are set out in Table 1. The experience to date from most BMT centers suggests that an oral dose of BU ranging between 14 and 16 mg/kg or 5 mg/kg dimethyl BU given intravenously in addition to 200 mg/kg CY is usually sufficient to eliminate the host's stem cells and immune system. The use of TBI for thalassemic stem cell ablation has not proved to give better results than chemotherapy with a combination of BU and CY.

This regimen would appear very satisfactory. Since the patients are young children, the possibility of secondary malignancies or developmental abnormalities after high-dose TBI must be considered seriously [6]. It should be noted that to date no malignancy has been reported in patients with nonmalignant disease prepared with chemotherapy alone [14].

Marrow Transplantation

Marrow is harvested by means of multiple aspiration from pelvic bones and, occasionally, from the sternum, with the donor under general anesthesia and under sterile conditions. Nucleated marrow cells – 4.1×10^8 per kilogram of the recipient's body weight (range $1.5–9.9 \times 10^8$ per kg) [7] – are then infused into the recipient intravenously. The infusion takes place 36 h after the last dose of CY and within 24 h of TBI, if performed.

Engraftment is determined by a change in the pattern of hemoglobin (Hb) synthesis (α/β-chain ratio), of Hb electrophoresis, and of red blood cell (RBC) antigens, and by cytogenetic analysis. The median duration for engraftment is 18 days (with a range of 7–55 days) [7].

Most of the patients were treated in positive pressure isolation rooms, and some of them in laminar airflow rooms [1]. They received oral nonabsorbable antibiotics and low-bacterial diet. Prophylactic systemic antibiotics, amikacin and piperacillin, were given on day 1 and continued until the granulocyte level exceeded 0.5×10^9/liter and the recipient was afebrile. Patients with persistent fever were treated with amphotericin B. Platelets were maintained at 20×10^9/liter with platelet transfusions, and the hematocrit (Hct) at 30% with RBC transfusions. Granulocyte transfusions were not given. All blood products were irradiated with 1.5–2.0 Gy.

Most centers use the following drugs alone or in various combinations for prevention of GVHD, which occurs in more than 53% of patients within the pediatric age group [8]: methotrexate (MTX, 10 mg/m^2), CY (7.5 mg/kg), and cyclosporin A (CSA, 5 mg/kg). In most patients, this regimen was discontinued after 6 months. More recently, the Jerusalem group has suggested that it is feasible to eliminate GVHD completely by removal of mature and committed T-lymphocytes from the donor marrow before transplantation using a new, immunoglobulin M, monoclonal rat (ant-human) lymphocyte-specific antibody, Campath 1, and donor serum as a source of complement. The major advantage of this method is that no postgrafting immunosuppression is required.

Results and Complications

Initially, Lucarelli et al treated patients in advanced phases of thalassemia major with CY and TBI. This conditioning regimen failed to eradicate the patient's stem cells even when 200 mg/kg CY and TBI of 8 Gy were used [9]. The use of a combination of BU, CY, and TBI of 30 Gy, although followed by successful engraftment, proved too toxic. Accordingly, Lucarelli et al. decided to modify the conditioning regimen to 14 mg/kg BU and 200 mg/kg CY. This was successful, and the results are summarized in Table 2. Patients were divided into two groups according to age, with 35 less than 8 years old (group 1) and 40 aged between 8 and 14 years (group 2).

In group 1, 26 (74%) of the patients were alive and free of thalassemia 3–31 months post transplantation, 4 (13%) were alive with thalassemia, and 5 (14%) had died. In group 2, 28 (70%) were alive and free of thalassemia 199-878 days post transplantation, 2 (5%) were alive with thalassemia, and 10 (25%) had died. Lin et al. [10] treated ten patients with a mean age of 6 years (range 1 year 7 months – 13 years): four survived free of thalassemia, four survived with thalassemia, and two died. In Pescara, di Girolamo et al. [11] treated 15 patients, 1–7 years old, of whom 13 survived free of thalassemia, 1 survived with thalassemia, and only 1 died.

Table 2. Results of BMT in two different age-groups [4, 7]

	Group 1	Group 2
No. of patients	35	40
No. of transfusions		
0– 10	11	-
10– 50	21	-
50–100	3	-
100–200	-	
Average	15	136 (range 60–180)
Regular desferrioxamine	13	13
Irregular desferrioxamine	-	27
Splenectomy	3	8
Hepatomegaly (2 cm)	11	38
Splenomegaly (2 cm)	9	25
Hepatitis Ag + Ab	14	1 + 18
Skeleton deformities	9	12
Heart disease	4	-
Condition post-BMT		
Alive	26 (74%)	28 (70%)
Alive with thalassemia	4 (13%)	2 (5%)
Dead	5 (14%)	10 (25%)
Acute GVHD	8 (23%)	11 (29%)
Chronic GVHD	2 (5%)	5 (12%)
Graft failure	6 (17%)	5 (13%)

Lucarelli's older group permits one to estimate the probability of developing acute GVHD: this was 29% (grade II or greater) [3] in patients with sustained first engraftment vs 23% in younger patients. Furthermore, the incidence of chronic GVHD was 12% in the older group vs 5% in the younger group.

Graft failure occurred in 5 (13%) of the patients in group 2. In two of them, thalassemic erythropoiesis recurred (within 33 and 311 days respectively), and the other three patients remained aplastic. In group 1, graft failure occurred in 6 (17%) of the patients, which is rather surprising. The average number of transfusions in the older group was 136, as compared with 15 in the younger group. The overall mortality in young patients was

14% [5], as compared with 25% [10] in the older group. The main causes of death were infections, interstitial pneumonia, acute GVHD, and myocardial failure.

Discussion

The major attempt to eradicate thalassemia major is by selective abortion after prenatal diagnosis using molecular biology techniques. Nevertheless, the estimated number of newborn homozygotes with thalassemia major all over the world is around 100 000 per year [12], and for Greece it is less than 40 per year.

Until new therapeutic approaches are used with success, such as insertion of normal β-genes into stem cells of patients with thalassemia major or activiation of γ-globin genes to encourage persistence of fetal HB into adult life, the current therapy for thalassemia major remains conventional treatment and BMT.

The possibility of a cure for thalassemia major by BMT creates a dilemma for patients, family, and physician. In practical terms, the overall benefits of BMT and the risk of early death from the procedure, even when irradiation is not used, must be compared with the effectiveness and disadvantages of current treatment. With transfusions and chelation therapy, life expectancy may exceed the age of 25 years; however, this regimen has many disadvantages and demands constant and expensive medical care. Usually splenectomy also becomes necessary, and long-term transfusion therapy is complicated by the development of multiple antibodies to red cell, leukocyte, and platelet antigens. On top of that, we also have the risk of transfusion-transmitted disease, mainly AIDS currently.

Based on the recent results from Italy (Pesaro, Pescara), BMT appears to be the treatment of choice in young patients with thalassemia major (if a suitable donor is available) from a purely medical point of view because of the potential cure and improved quality of life it may offer. BMT for thalassemia does not seem so expensive (around U.S.$ 10000 in Pesaro, paid only once) set against an adequate transfusion regimen, with its yearly cost of between U.S.$ 5000 and 20000 during the patients's whole life.

Summary

If a suitable donor is available, bone marrow transplantation is feasible in patients with thalassemia major aged from 6 months to 15 years and offers the hope of curing this congenital disorder.

References

1. Thomas ED, Buckner CD, Sanders JE et al. (1982) Marrow transplantation for talassemia. Lancet ii: 227–229
2. Lucarelli G, Izzi T, Polchi P. et al. (1983) Trapianto di midollo osseo nella talassemia. Transfus Sangue 1:62-64
3. Lucarelli G. Galimberti M, Polchi P. et al (1986) Marrow transplantation in patients with advanced thalassemia. Blood 68: 275
4. Lucarelli G, Polchi P, Galimberti M, et al. (1987) Bone marrow transplantation in thalassemia. In: Sirchia G, Zanella A (eds) Thalassemia today, the Mediterranean experience. Milan
5. Clift RA, Hansen JA, Thomas ED et al. (1979) Marrow transplantation from donors other than HLA-identical silbings. Transplantation 28:235-242
6. Slavin S and EA Rachmilewitz (1986) Bone marrow transplantation in thalassemia. Bone Marrow Transplant 1: 11–15
7. Lucarelli G, Polchi P, Galiberti M et al. (1985) Marrow transplantation for thalassemia following Busulphan and cyclophosphamide. Lancet ii: 1355–1357
8. O'Reilly RJ, Brochstein J, Dinsmore R, Kirkpatrick D (1984) Marrow transplantation for congenital disorders. Semin Hematol 21: 188–221
9. Lucarelli G, Polchi P, Izzi T, et al. (1984). Allogeneic marrow transplantation for thalassemia. Exp Hematol 12: 676
10. Lin KH, Lin KS, Feig SA (1986). Marrow transplantation for thalassemia, Bone Marrow Transplantation 1: 115–120

11. Girolamo G, di Bartolomeo P, Angrilli F et al. (1987). Bone marrow transplantation for refractory anaemia and congenital haemopathies (thalassemias, chronic granulomatous disease, Fanconi's disease). XIII annual meeting of the EBMT Interlaken, Switzerland, 1-5 March 1987 (Abstr 43).
12. Anonymous (1981) Community control of hereditary anaemias (Memorandum). Bull WHO, 61: 63
13. Thomas ED (1985) Marrow transplantation for non malignant disorders. N Engl Med 312: 46–47
14. Sullivan MK, Joachim Deeg H, Sanders EJ et al (1984). Late complications after marrow transplantation. Semin Hematol 21: 1

16 Partial Splenic Embolization in the Management of Thalassemia

C. Politis and D. G. Spigos

Introduction

Thalassemia becomes complicated by hypersplenism in any patient at some time during the clinical course, and this leads to a progressive increase of transfusional requirements [1]. Splenectomy usually results in a substantial decline of transfusional needs. Unfortunately, the effectiveness of splenectomy is not easily predictable. About 1 year after the operation, a small proportion of splenectomized thalassemic patients have again increased transfusional needs. Furthermore, the risk of overwhelming postsplenectomy infection is higher in these patients than in many other groups of splenectomized individuals [2, 3]. Hypoxemia with pulmonary artery embolism has also been reported after splenectomy in thalassemic patients [4].

From the surgical point of view, splenectomy is not always safe for those thalassemic patients with special clinical problems, such as cardiac failure, liver cirrhosis, and diabetes. For these reasons, alternatives to splenectomy have been attempted in recent years, such as partial splenic embolization (PSE) [5] and partial vascular disconnection of the spleen [6].

Transcatheter arterial embolization of the spleen has gained increased acceptance in the treatment of various conditions with hypersplenism [7]. In 1973, for the first time, Maddison [8] successfully performed arterial embolization of the spleen in an attempt to eliminate hypersplenism. This procedure was subsequently abandoned because of a high incidence of complications, such as splenic abscess and splenic rupture, causing death in many cases. In 1979, partial ablation of the splenic mass was performed by Spigos et al. [9] in an immunosuppressed renal allograft recipient. The success of this operation encouraged them to extend the procedure electively to a small group of patients with indications for splenectomy.

The results of a prospective randomized study comparing transcatheter PSE with splenectomy in renal transplant candidates demonstrated that PSE offers an acceptably safe alternative to splenectomy in patients in whom both surgical intervention and the resulting asplenic state carry a prohibitive risk [9].

Given these encouraging results, PSE has been extended to a group of hypersplenic patients with thalassemia in an effort to reduce transfusional requirements while preserving splenic immune function [5]. Seven patients with thalassemia major (three males and four females), 9–22 years of age, and one male patient with thalassemia intermedia, 48 years of age, underwent PSE by Politis et al. [5] (Table 1). All patients were candidates for splenectomy on the basis of hypersplenism: they presented with a large spleen and required transfusion at 14–21 day intervals to maintain a hemoglobin (Hb) level of about 10 g/100 ml. Leukocyte and platelet counts were normal in all but one, who had severe leukopenia and thrombocytopenia, suffering from frequent rhinorrhagias and infections [5]. These results were compared with those for a group of patients who had undergone splenectomy [5].

Table 1. The proportion of spleen embolized in each of the thalassemic patients treated with partial splenic embolization

Patient no.	Sex	Age at PSE (years)	% PSE	Follow-up (years)
1	F	13	30 (1st PSE) 70 (Total)	1
2	F	9	85	1
3	M	15	90	6
4	M	21	60	6
5	F	22	90	6
6	M	9	70	3
7	F	14	70	1 ½
8	M	48	20 (1st PSE) 40 (Total)	1 ½

Procedure

The technique used has already been reported [5]. Each patient receives a providone-iodine bath the night before and on the morning of the embolization and also receives appropriate doses of either gentamycin and penicillin or cefamandole nafate immediately before being transferred for angiography.

An epidural anesthetic with bupivacaine hydrochloride (0,5%) is used to achieve a sensory level of T4 in order to block the sympathetic pain fibers from the spleen. Narcotic sedation has occasionally been given to patients who suffered severe pain during the procedure, and to another adult with thalassemia intermedia and serious clinical problems (enormous splenomegaly, liver damage, cardiopathy, and alloimmunization).

The splenic artery is selectively catheterized via a percutaneous femoral artery approach. A basal angiogram is obtained, and the spleen is embolized with up to 40 pieces of absorbable gelfoam pledgets. The extent of infarction is monitored fluoroscpically and confirmed on completion of the procedure by a second angiogram. Prior to discharge, a liver-spleen scan is obtained to confirm the extent of the infarction. Angiographic estimates of infarction size agree closely with those found on the liver-spleen scan (Figs. 1, 2). In all but two cases, 70%–90% of the splenic mass was infarcted (Table 1) [5].

All the patients are treated with desferrioxamine. They are vaccinated against pneumococcus (Pneumovax) prior to the procedure and are maintained on long-term prophylactic penicillin.

Immediate Postoperative Follow-Up

According to Politis et al. [5], only one of seven patients presented severe pain, which lasted 48 h, whereas all the other patients did well without marked pain. All the patients ran a "pseudoseptic" episode for the first postembolization day, with mild fever, elevated leukocyte count, and enlargement of the spleen (Fig. 3). Four patients developed pleural effusions (none of which required thoracocentesis), and two had some degree of left lower lobe atelectasis. Mild leukocytosis and thrombocytosis were demonstrated in most patients.

The increase in platelet and leukocyte numbers in all of the patients reached its peak in the first 2 weeks after embolization (mean leukocyte count, 13 000/mm^3; mean platelet count, 400 000/mm^3). The increase was transient, and the counts returned to normal within 6 months. In patient 1, the preexisting

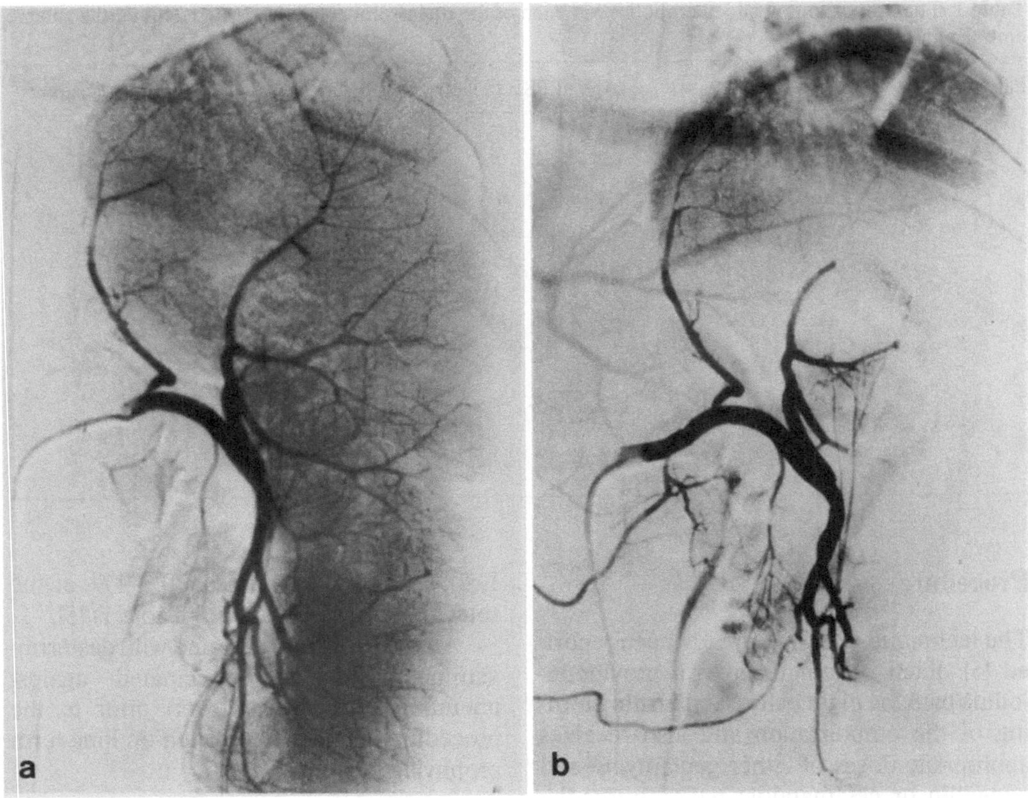

Fig. 1 a, b. Preembolization (**a**) and postembolization (**b**) spleen angiograms (arterial phase). An estimated 90% of the spleen has been embolized

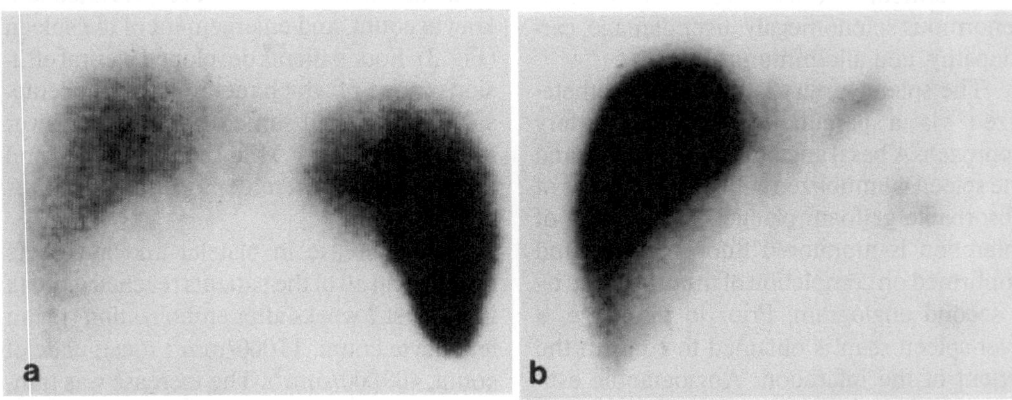

Fig. 2a,b. Preembolization (**a**) and postembolization (**b**) liver-spleen scans (anterior view) of patient in Fig. 1. An estimated 90% of the spleen has been embolized

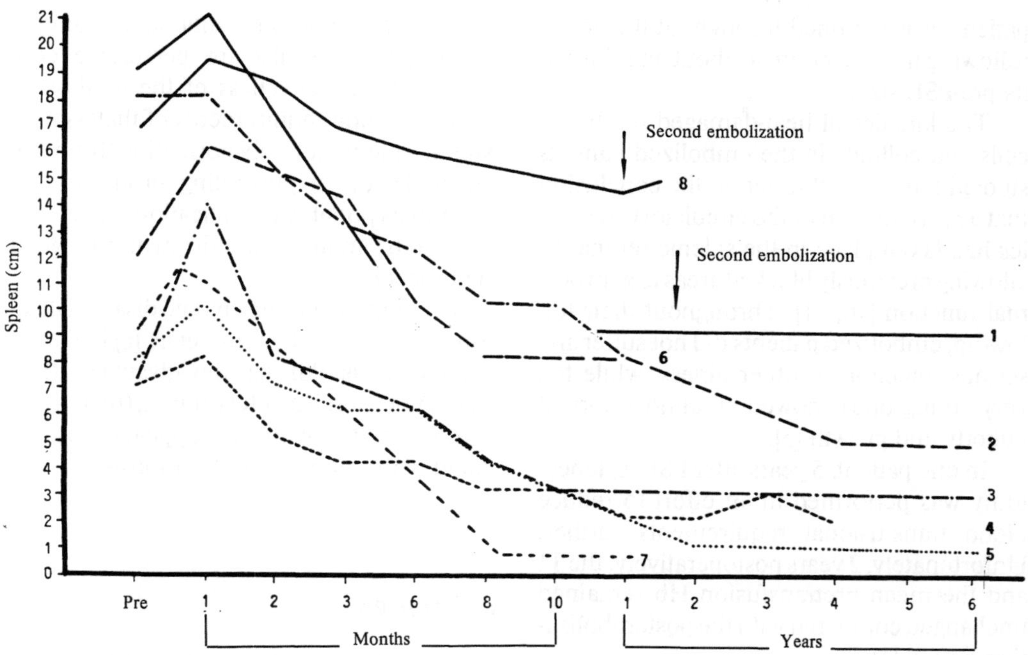

Fig. 3. Changes of spleen size prior to and following PSE [5]

leukopenia and thrombocytopenia were corrected after the first PSE [5].

Immediately after PSE, all patients presented a slight increase of circulating erythroblasts (range 12–46/100 leukocytes), which were stabilized a few months later at a lower level (range 10–35/100 leukocytes) [5]. Leukocytosis subsided gradually during the following months, while the platelet and erythroblasts counts still remained at the same high level (mean platelet count, 632 140/ mm^3; erythroblasts range, 48-233/100 leukocytes) [5].

Long-Term Follow-Up

A statistically significant change ($p<0.001$) of the transfusion index (TI)[1] value was observed in the two PSE and splenectomy groups of patients immediately after the procedure; it remained unchanged thereafter. Changes of mean Hb level were not significant in either group, although a steady, slight increase had been recorded during the years after PSE. No significant differences existed between the two groups concerning the above parameters, either prior to or after the procedures [5].

A statistically significant difference was observed only in the case of immunoglobulin M the level of which remained significantly higher ($p<0.005$) in the embolized patients than in the splenectomized group during the overall period of their follow-up [5].

In both groups, which had about the same ferritin level prior to the procedures, an increase of 68% was observed during the 1st subsequent year. In the following years, ferritin levels gradually declined in both groups, now being significantly lower in all patients than prior to the procedure ($p<0.01$).

A significant prolongation ($p=0.025$) of red cell survival was detected in the embolized patients 1 year after PSE (mean t1/2 increase, 5.64 days). The spleen of embolized

[1] $$TI = \frac{\text{milliliters of blood per day per sq. m. of body surface}}{\text{mean Hb}}$$

patients was confined throughout the years following the procedure to about one-third of its pre-PSE size.

The kinetics of heat-damaged red blood cells and colloids in the embolized patients studied long after PSE led to the conclusion that a reorientation of the circulatory dynamics had taken place in the splenic remnants, allowing previously blocked areas to gain normal function [10, 11]. Throughout their follow-up, embolized patients did not suffer any serious infection or other illness, while the very young ones showed an almost normal puberty and growth [5].

In one patient, 5 years after PSE, splenectomy was performed in an effort to reduce blood transfusional requirements further. Unfortunately, 2 years postoperatively, the TI and the mean pretransfusion Hb remained unchanged compared with the postembolization period [5].

The most striking amelioration in the clinical and hematological picture was observed in the adult with thalassemia intermedia. The embolization of even a small proportion of the enormous spleen of this patient caused a remarkable improvement 1 year after the procedure, at which time a second embolization was applied, resulting in further improvement [5].

As for the group of splenectomized controls, two of these patients presented with recurrent infections [5].

Comment

In recent years, alternatives to operative splenectomy have been sought in the management of thalassemia that might offer the advantages of such a surgical intervention without its high risks. PSE has proved to be a safe and relatively easy procedure to perform. The results of the 1- to 7-year follow-up of 7 patients indicate that, in the management of thalassemia, PSE is a reliable alternative to splenectomy. Immediate post-PSE results are reassuring as regards the safety of the procedure. Morever, PSE represents a relatively easy procedure of interventional radiology.

Long-term results are persuasive concerning the effectiveness of the method in reducing blood requirements of thalassemic patients and in not only correcting thrombocytopenia but also preventing thrombocythemia and its possible complications. This may prove to be another signifficant advantage of the procedure.

In comparison with splenic disarterialization as performed by Girot et al. [6] in thalassemic patients, PSE has the advantages that: (a) it is not a surgical intervention, (b) it can be repeated, and (c) it does not appear to be associated with splenic vein thrombosis.

References

1. Modell B, Berdoukas V (1984) The clinical approach to thalssemia. Grune and Stratton, New York
2. Smith CH, Erlandson ME, Stern G, Hilgartner MW (1964) Postsplenectomy infection in Cooley's anemia. Ann NY Acad Sci 119: 748–757
3. Eraklis AJ, Kevy SV, Diamond LK, Cross RE (1967) Hazard of overwhelming infection after splenectomy in childhood. N Engl J Med 276: 1225–1229
4. Fucharoen S (1981) Hypoxaemia and the effect of aspirin in thalassemia. Southeast Asian J Trop Med Public Health 12: 90–93
5. Politis C, Spigos DG, Georgiopoulou P, Vrettou H, Economidou J, Germenis A, Richardson C, Papaevangelou G (1987) Partial splenic embolization for hypersplenism of thalassemia major. Five year follow-up. Br Med J 294: 665–667
6. Girot R, Revillon Y, Barritault L, Gire R, Beringer A, Boiteux F(1984) Hypersplenisme de la thalassémie majeure. Traitement par désartérialisation partielle de la rate. Résultats préliminaires à propos de 5 cas. Presse Med 13: 1881
7. Mozes MF, Spigos DG, Pollak R, Abejo R, Pavel DG, Tan WS, Jonasson O (1984) Partial splenic embolization, an alternative to splenectomy results of a prospective randomized study. Surgery 96: 694–702
8. Maddison FE (1973) Embolic therapy of hypersplenism. Invest Radiol 8: 280–281
9. Spigos DG, Jonasson O, Mozes M, Capek V (1979) Partial splenic embolization in the treatment of hypersplenism. Am J Radiol 132: 777–782

10. Germenis A, Dimitriou P, Kasfiki A, Antipas SE (1986) Kinetics of heat-damaged homologous red blood cells in patients with homozygous β-thalassemia in relation to blood transfusion. Scand J Haematol 36: 450–456

11. Germenis A, Antipas SE, Dimitriou P, Politis C, Spigos DG (1988) Assessment of splenic and RES function of patients with thalassemia major long after partial splenic embolisation: In vivo clearance study. Eur J Hematol 40: 466–472

17 Ultrasound-Guided Procedures for Prenatal Diagnosis of Hemoglobinopathies

A. Antsaklis

Introduction

Prenatal diagnosis of various congenital abnormalities and inherited diseases, with selective termination of affected pregnancies, has been universally accepted and extensively applied for the last 15 years [1, 2]. In particular, prenatal diagnosis of hemoglobinopathies including thalassemia is generally performed by globin chain synthesis studies on fetal blood samples obtained by fetoscopic or ultrasound-guided techniques in the second trimester of pregnancy [3, 4], or by DNA analysis of chorionic villi samples obtained by ultrasound-guided techniques in the first trimester of pregnancy [5, 6]. Ultrasound scanning plays a central role in enhancing the safety and effectiveness of these diagnostic procedures.

Fetoscopy-Guided Procedure for Fetal Blood Sampling

Valenti [7] described the endoamnioscope, a modification of a pediatric cystoscope, 6.8 mm in diameter, and a year later, using the same endoscope, Valenti was the first to describe a technique for obtaining blood samples from the vessels of the umbilical cord during laparotomy [8]. These pregnancies were interrupted by hysterotomy immediately after endoscopy.

Hobbins and Mahoney [9] and Patrick et al. [10] were the first to describe a technique for obtaining fetal blood samples with a 1.7-mm-diameter Needlescope, using a local anesthetic. Since 1974, the technique of obtaining fetal blood samples under festoscopic direct visualization has been applied by several groups investigators in various parts of the world [11]. The current data on fetoscopy quitted fetal blood sampling experience, collected at the Eighth International Fetoscopy Group Meeting in Rotterdam 1986 [12], is given in Table 1.

A program for fetal blood sampling by fetoscopy requires genetic counselors and clinicans with experience in fetoscopy and ultrasound, while successful blood sampling depends on the operator's experience. Before the procedure, the patients must have appropriate genetic counseling - including a discussion of the indications, possibilities, and limitations of the technique - so that they may give informed consent.

One of the first considerations in establishing a fetoscopy program is wheter a demand exists in a community.

For this reason the ethnic background of the community, rather than its size, may be important. In Greece, the mean incidence of β-thalassemia carriers ranges between 2.3% and 14%, and is one of the countries where prenatal diagnosis of β-thalassemia by fetal blood sampling was rapidly applied on a large scale because of the high prevalence and considerable impact of this disease [13].

The optimum stage of gestation for obtaining fetal blood is after the 18th week of pregnancy. Before the 18th week, the fetus is small relative to the volume of amniotic fluid, and its total blood volume is not great enough to compensate for an acute blood loss of 1-2 ml [14]. The vessels of the fetal placental surface before the 18th week of pregnancy are also small, so that puncturing and blood withdrawal is difficult. After the 20th week of

Table 1. Current data on obstetical procedures for prenatal diagnosis

Procedure	No. of Centers	No. of patients	Selective termination	Fetal losses		Continuing pregnancies	Children born and survived
				Before 28 weeks	After 28 weeks		
Fetoscopy and FBS	12	5189	1299	181	29	235	3428
Placentocentesis and FBS	5	375	99	25	1	13	237
Cordocentesis and FBS	17	468	90	15	34	126	208
CVS							
Transvervical catheter	47	13124	726	182	0	5688	6525
Transcervical biopsy forceps	8	1445	255	101	31	435	724
Transabdominal needle aspiration	7	862	35	20	1	445	361

Data were reported at the Eigth Annual Meeting of the International Fetoscopy Group, Rotterdam, September 1986. FBS: fetal blood sampling

pregnancy, visibility within the amniotic cavity is decreased significantly due to increased turbidity of the amniotic fluid and increased size of the fetus, uterus, and placenta [11].

Instrumentarium

A fetoscope widely used for obtaining fetal blood samples is the Dyonics Needlescope. This fetoscope is a fiber-optic system with a source of cold light. The fetoscope is an inflexible endoscope, 1.7 mm in diameter and 155 mm long [15] (Fig. 1–3).

Operative Technique

Ultrasound scanning is performed before fetoscopy to determine gestational age; the exact size of the placenta, as well as its thickness and margins; the position of the fetus within the amniotic cavity; the site of insertion of the umbilical cord on the placenta; and a site for inserting the fetoscope. Fetoscopy performed under real-time ultrasound guidance may assist the fetoscopist during the procedure; however, the maneuvers of the probe often impede manipulation of the fetoscope.

A vessel situated a few centimeters from the insertion site of the umbilical cord is chosen for blood sampling (Fig. 4). Pure fetal blood can be taken from an umbilical cord vessel at the site of its insertion into the placenta [16–18]. Placental location, amniotic fluid turbidity, and multiple pregnancy constitute special problems for fetal blood sampling [19–21].

Nonfetoscopic Procedures for Fetal Blood Sampling

Placentocentesis

Preparation of the patient for placentocentesis is similar to that required for fetoscopy. Ultrasound is used to determine the location of the placenta, its margins, and a site for needle insertion. A 19 gauge needle is inserted without ultrasound guidance through the abdominal wall into the amniotic cavity. Puncturing of a vessel on the fetal placental surface causes bleeding into the amniotic cavity [22]. Care must be taken to avoid punc-

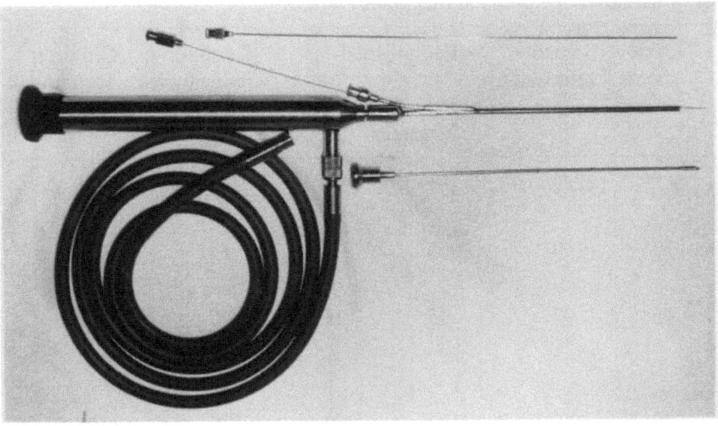

Fig. 1. The fetoscope

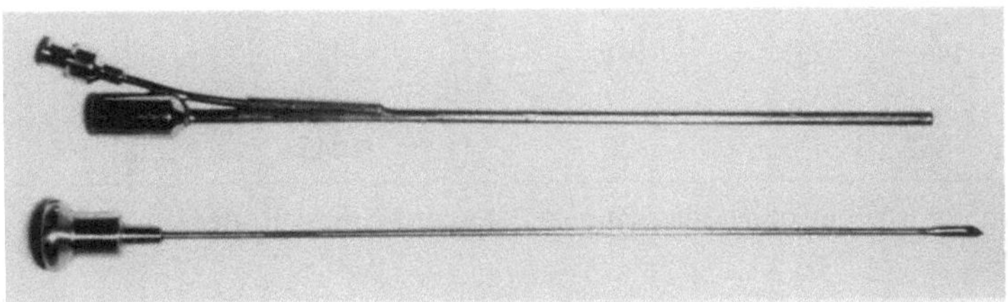

Fig. 2. The special Y cannula with trocar for fetal blood sampling

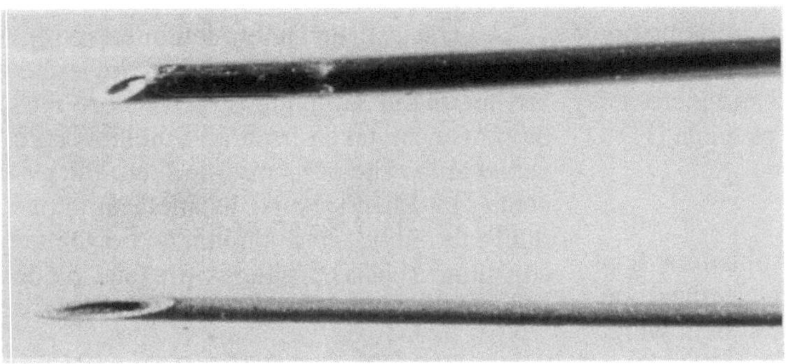

Fig. 3. Special needles tapered at the end for pure fetal blood sampling

turing any of the large fetal vessels in the area of cord insertion. The samples of blood-stained amniotic fluid are immediately analyzed with a Coulter counter for the presence of fetal blood. If no fetal red blood cells are found, another puncture of the placenta is attempted at a different site. No agreement exists about the number of attempts that should be made. In 10%–20% of cases, the procedure has to be repeated one or more times before a sample with even a small percentage of fetal cells is obtained [23].

Ultrasound-Guided Cordocentesis

The technique of ultrasound-guided cordecentesis has been tried to combine the simplicity of placentocentesis with the efficiency of fetoscopy in order to obtain pure fetal blood samples. Under continuous sector real-time ultrasound guidance, a 21-gauge needle - 10–13 cm long, filled with a 3.8% sodium citrate solution and fixed to a 0.2-ml disposable syringe containing 0.1 ml of this solution - is introduced transabdominally and advanced toward the umbilical cord vein.

This vein is punctured at about 1 cm from the placental insertion. The advancement of the needle is followed on the oscilloscope by a clearly visible echo, emitted by the needle tip (Fig. 5). In case of an anterior placenta, the needle is introduced transplacentally [24], avoiding introduction into the amniotic cavity (Fig. 5b).

Immediately after the first drop of blood has been obtained, the syringe is changed and replaced by a new one containing no additive. The blood sample is immediately transferred into special tubes containing adequate anticoagulant. The current data on cordocentesis, collected at the Eighth International Fetoscopy Group Meeting, are given in Table 1 [12].

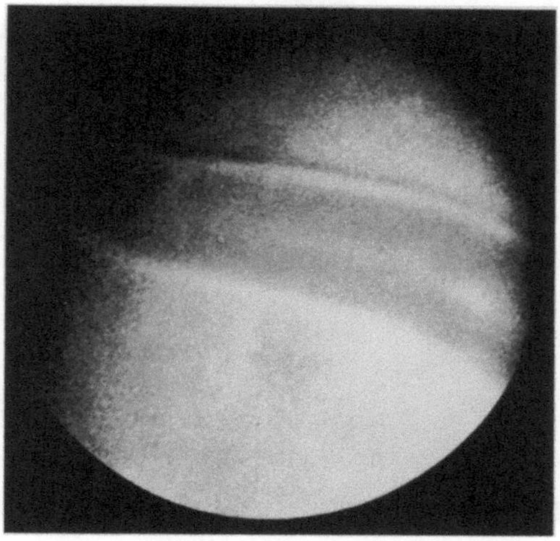

Fig. 4. Fetoscopic view of chorionic plate vessel

Chorionic Villi Sampling

Prenatal diagnosis of hemoglobinopathies, as previously reported, is generally performed by globin chain synthesis studies on fetal blood obtained by fetoscopic or ultrasound-guided techniques in the second trimester of pregnancy. These techniques have proved to be safe and diagnostically accurate only after the 18th week of gestation. However, because prenatal diagnosis in the second trimester involves both medical and psychological problems, the aim of several investigators in recent years has been to make prenatal diagnosis possible earlier in pregnancy [25, 26].

Amniotic fluid cells have been found to be most appropriate for these studies on the feasibility of genetic mapping of the DNA extracted from this material, which proved to be a major breakthrough in further developing first-trimester prenatal diagnosis. Trophoblast DNA has recently been used for prenatal diagnosis of inherited hemoglobinopathies [5, 6, 27]. The detection of β-thalassemia mutations by DNA analysis in a fetus at risk can be achieved by either direct or indirect assays, or by the use of synthetic oligonucleotides [29, 30]. The main advantage of this method is that chorionic villi may be obtained at an early stage of gestation, which may make prenatal diagnosis a more acceptable procedure for an increasing number of couples at risk.

In recent years, application of prenatal diagnosis in the first trimester of pregnancy has spread rapidly and successfully in several centers. In April 1983, only eight of them, including the center in Athens, were able to report their diagnostic experience on a limited number of females at risk. In September 1985, the mailing list of the International Chorionic Villi Sampling (CVS) Collaborative Study contained more than 80 centers in Europe and North America, with a total experience of about 9,000 diagnostic cases. CVS has been attempted using several approaches and apparatuses. On the whole, there are four main methods: (a) CVS by direct vision, (b) CVS by "blind" aspiration, (c) CVS under ultrasound guidance, and (d) transabdominal CVS. These will be discussed in the following sections, where detailed description of the techniques in current use will preceded by an account of their development over the last decade. The advantages of first-trimester fetal diagnosis compared with blood sampling by fetoscopy can be seen in Table 1 [31–34]. In summary, the advantages of CVS are:

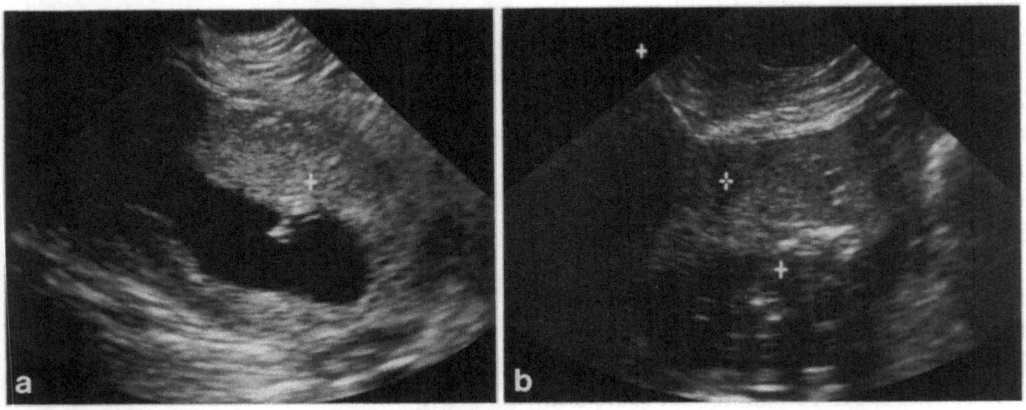

Fig. 5 a, b. Transplacental access and fetal blood sampling from the cord vessels (see text)

1. It reduces the waiting period.
2. It produces less social and psychological stress.
3. It permits earlier and safer therapeutic abortion.
4. It allows couples "privacy", as pregnancies not yet obvious.

Role of Ultrasound in CVS

Ultrasound scanning has a central role in enhancing the safety and effectiveness of CVS [35]. The initial ultrasound scanning, usually carried out at the first counseling session, will give information on the viability of fetus, the yolk sac, umbilical cord insertion, placental site, and gestational age. The developing placenta is easily identified as a uniformly hyperechoic area along a portion of the gestational sac. Between the 8th and 11th week of gestation, the cross-sectional diameter of the thickest portion of the chorion frondosum varies from 8 to 15 mm. This information is confirmed prior to CVS. Ultrasound visualization of the bladder functions as an acoustic window to the uterus and its contents; in addition, it severes to keep the corpo-cervical junction straight. However, overfilling of the bladder may cause technical problems during the procedure [36].

CVS has been attempted using several approaches and apparatuses, and the most widely applied ultrasound-guided techniques are as follows:

1. Transcervical
   a) Catheter aspiration
   b) Biopsy forceps
2. Transabdominal: needle aspiration

Transcervical Techniques

Transcervical CVS under ultrasound guidance can be carried out with suction into a thin tube or by biopsy with a suitable forceps. Both techniques have their own merits and drawbacks and have been widely applied over the last 2 years.

CVS by Catheter Aspiration

More than 60% of investigators around the world are using the transcervical aspiration technique. The plastic catheter used (Portex Ltd., UK) consists of a polyethylene tube with an external diameter of 1.5 mm of which one end is moulded to fit a syringe and the other is rounded (Fig. 6). The length of the catheter varies from 21 to 26 cm.

Technique

On starting the procedure, an ultrasound examination is performed with the patient's bladder partially filled, so that the exact site of

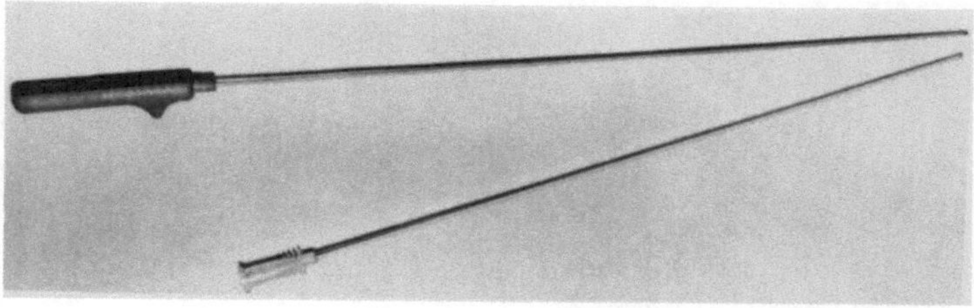

Fig. 6. The Portex plastic catheter with soft obturator which fits into it

chorion frondosum and umbilical cord insertion can be located. The patient is placed in the lithotomy position. Using a speculum, the cervix is visualized, and the anterior lip is grasped with a toothed tenaculum. The pinch sometimes causes mild pain to the patient, this being the only discomfort throughout the whole procedure. Subsequently, the uterine position is again evaluated by ultrasound, and the sampling catheter is slowly inserted through the cervix under ultrasound guidance. Both operators - sonographer and sampler - need a three-dimensional view of the uterine cavity so that they can coordinate their movements in guiding the tip of the catheter. At this point, it is important that no resistance be felt, and that the cannula tip be visualized continuously on the screen. Blind introduction of the catheter could cause trauma and pain. To straighten the cervical canal, the cervix may have to be pulled slightly. The tip of the catheter is directed to the sampling site by the appropriate manipulations. The ideal placement is well into the placental substance, away from the decidua and about 1 mm away from the gestation sac.

Entering the amniotic sac is undesirable; should this occur, the catheter is pulled gently backward. When the tip of the catheter lies against the decidua, sampling by suction should be avoided, as it may open maternal sinuses and lead to excessive bleeding. For the same reason, sampling close to the insertion of the cord should also be avoided, although some investigators have used this area as a target, especially when carrying out CVS on twins.

When the correct position of the catheter is confirmed, the operator carefully removes the obturator and attaches a 20 ml syringe to the end of the catheter. The syringe contains 2–3 ml of an appropriate culture medium. Following that, a negative pressure of 5–10 ml is applied. This is adequate to cause sucking of several villous tips into the cannula, where they are ultrasonically visible. Subsequently, the catheter with the syringe is pulled slightly backward to detach the sample, the negative pressure is gradually released, and the system gently removed. The obtained sample is flushed gently under sterile conditions into a plastic petri dish. The procedure does not require premedication or any other preparations. Slight spotting may occur up to 48 h after the procedure. Pregnant women are asked to have an ultrasound examination within the following 7 days in order to confirm the smooth progress of pregnancy [1, 39].

CVS by Biopsy Forceps

Attempts to obtain chorionic villi using a biopsy forceps under ultrasound guidance were first reported in 1982 by a Soviet group [35]. In 1983, Goosens et al. [27] reported CVS under ultrasound guidance for preventing homozygous hemoglobin (Hb)S. Two years later, the total experience of this group extended over 120 uselected pregnancies, with a 100% rate of success in obtaining trophoblastic tissue and a 90% proportion of pure samples. Of the last 70 cases, none was followed by fetal loss. The authors reported that the number of forceps insertions necessary to yield a satisfactory sample and the frequency of miscarriages decreased as the operators acquired more experience with the technique [40]. The forceps is 30 cm long and has a diameter of 1,7 mm. It is rigid and easy to sterilize.

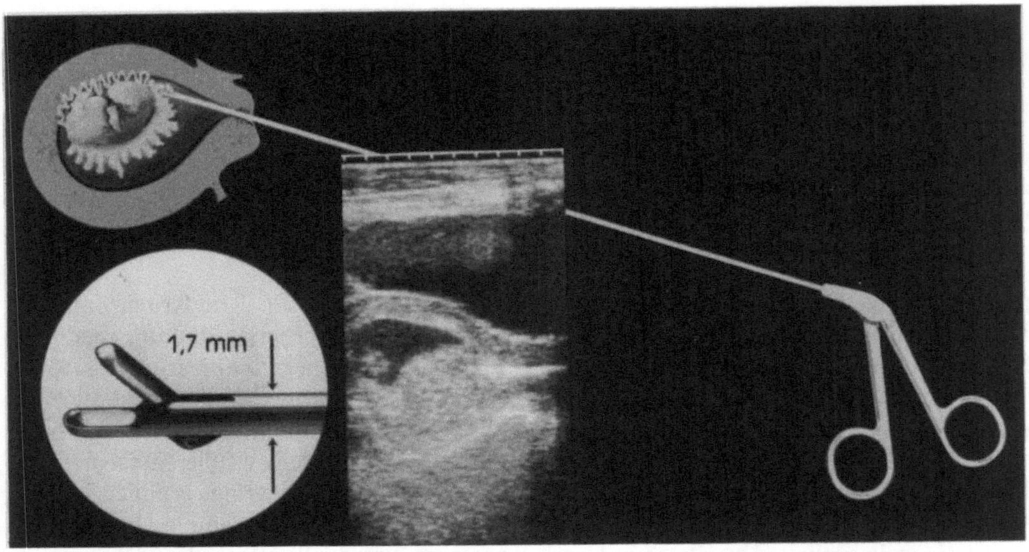

Fig. 7. Biopsy forceps technique. The *left inset* shows the forceps and the opening of the jaws, which can be easily visualized on the ultrasound screen *(right inset)*

An interesting feature is the design of its tip, which, when closed, is smooth and rounded and can be introduced atraumatically through the cervix. The opening of the jaws is large enough to be seen on the ultrasound screen and to grasp an adequate piece of trophoblast (Fig. 7).

Technique

The procedure can be carried out by a single operator on an outpatient basis without premidication or anesthesia. After the preliminary ultrasound examination, the patient is placed in the lithotomy position, the cervix is grasped with a tenaculum, and the closed biopsy forceps is inserted slowly through it under ultrasound guidance to the thickest zone of the trophoblast, very close to the chorionic plate. While being moved slowly forward, the forceps is opened. After that, its jaws are closed again, grasping firmly pieces of chorionic villi, which are detached on withdrawal and washed under sterile conditions in a petri dish.

Transabdominal Needle Aspiration Technique

The following alternative approach was reported in 1984 by Smidt-Jensen et al. [41]. The patient is placed in a supine position. The predetermined needle pathway is monitored by a sharp, stillette-point 17-gauge guide needle attached to the transducer head and follows a line parallel to the chorionic membranes. The most successful combination of needles is a sharp, stilette-pointed 17-gauge guide cannula and an inner 19-gauge aspirating needle, 1.5 cm longer than the guide needle. The guide needle is introduced through the abdominal wall and uterus until its tip can be seen on the screen just within the chorion frondosum. The stilette is then replaced with a 19-gauge aspirating needle, to which a 20 ml syringe has been attached. Since this needle is 1.5 cm longer than the guide, its tip is seen well within the chorion frondosum. Suction on the syringe combined with a gentle up-and-down movement allows collection of a sample. The chorionic villi are aspirated into heparinized Hank's buffered saline solution through repeated aspirations.

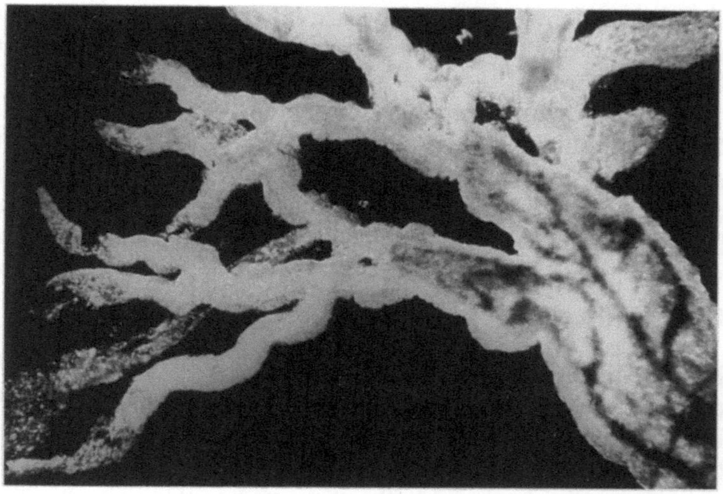

Fig. 8. Chorionic villi under low-power magnification (x 10)

A great advantage of the transabdominal procedure is that it is more acceptable to the patient since it is very similar to amniocentesis; moreover, it is more easily learned than the transcervical procedures [42].

Sample Processing

The aspirated chorionic villi are examined under an inverted or dissecting microscope by the attendant physician, who confirms the quality and quantity of the sample and separates it from maternal tissues inadvertently aspirated [28]. The chorionic villi have a distinotive appearance (Fig. 8). The quantity usually aspirated varies from a few villi up to 30 mg tissue. This is adequate for DNA studies (10-20 mg tissue may yield the necessary 10-20 μg DNA) and more than enough for direct cytogenetic analysis (usually 5-10 mg wet tissue suffices). If inadequate tissue is obtained, as many as three further attempts may be made with no significant increase in the risk of complications.

Technical Difficulties

The main technical difficulties in CVS are: (a) visualization of the sampling device, (b) uterine position and fibroids, and (c) multiple pregnancy.

One of the most frequent problems is the inability of the operator to detect by ultrasound the plastic tip of the catheter, which may be dislodged from the position set earlier under ultrasound guidance when the metallic obturator is removed from the cannula or when suction with the syringe is applied. This dislodgement increases the risk of sampling decidua and hence, the probability of failure and/or miscarriage. To increase echogenicity of the catheters, Holzgreve and Miny developed a new plastic catheter containing highly echogenic substances (20% barium sulfate), the use of which was associated with a decrease both in the number of insertions required to obtain an adequate sample and in the frequency of complications [43].

Another common technical difficulty in CVS is the occurrence of a steep uterine anteflexion with an anterior implantation site, or of a retroflexion with a posterior or fundal implantation site. Regulation of bladder fullness, cervical traction, and occasional uterine manipulations can be of help. However, the uterus is a dynamic organ and changes its shape by virtue of multiple contractions. Contractions may even change the entire orientation of the uterus from an anteflexed to a retroflexed position. Fibroids may create two problems: (a) distortion of the passageway and (b) increased distance between the implantation site and the cervical os. Both problems prevent the catheter from reaching the chorion.

Sampling a twin pregnancy is undoubtedly more difficult and dangerous than sampling a singleton pregnancy. In such cases, the cord insertion sites are used as target points for CVS.

Complications

In assessing the usefulness of a new medical procedure, it is important to know whether it is acceptable to the members of the population in which it will be applied.

As usually happens with each new method, CVS in the first trimester of pregnancy has not been spared a series of problems and risks resultung in fetal loss. World experience with CVS indicates a fetal loss rate of about 5% - 6% [44]. However, recent unpublished data on large series give figures ranging between only 2% and 5% [45]. These figures must be corrected for a host of confounding variables, such as: (a) maternal history of prior induced abortions, (b) maternal age, (c) gravidity, (d) environmental factors, and (e) paternal cytogenetic factors [46]. Fetal losses following CVS are not necessarily a result of it: during the first trimester of pregnancy, a large number of nonviable gestations result in miscarriage. Cytogenetic studies of these abortuses have shown that in at least 50% of cases serious chromosomal defects are present. Carrying out CVS in such cases would inevitably increase both the rate of fetal losses associated with the procedure and the incidence of lost fetuses with chromosomal defects. Obstetrical complications associated with CVS are summarized in Table 2.

Table 2. Complications after chorionic villi sampling

1. Perforation of the gestation sac
2. Infections
3. ABO-Rh isoimmunization
4. Vaginal bleeding
5. Spontaneous abortion

Perforation of the gestational sac has been the most frequent and serious complication when CVS was performed blind or using poor ultrasound apparatus [39, 47]. This complication rarely occurs today.

Another serious complication following CVS is the risk of infection since transcervical manipulations may readily contaminate the uterine cavity. Although it has not been well known that uterine infection is responsible for some of the fetal loses observed after CVS, a few cases of acute infection have been reported. So far, no relationship has been demonstrated between quantity of cervical flora and fetal loss. It has been recommended that the CVS catheter be used only once since it is difficult to maintain the sterility of a catheter when withdrawing it from the vagina once the obturator has been removed. It has been reported that the transabdominal route reduces the risk of intrauterine infection [41].

Vaginal bleeding may appear up to 10 days after the procedure and arises from the site where the chorionic villi were obtained. A slight vaginal bleeding may also occur from the site where the cervix is grasped during the procedure. To prevent this minor problem, some obstetricians manage to avoid using the tenaculum.

The incidence of complications is related to the quality of the ultrasound equipment, the number of attempts, the gestational age, and the experience of the obstetrician. It has been recommended that no more than two catheter insertions be performed. It has also been reported that CVS by the transcervical route has a very high abortion rate in comparison with the transabdominal route [41]. Several centers in the world. (Milan, Chicago, Philadelphia) [45] with extensive experience in diagnostic CVS using the transcervical route had cumulative fetal loss rates of 2.3% in 353 pregnancies. These results compare favorably with the substantial diagnostic series using the transabdominal route in which Hahnemann reported a 2.86% fetal loss rate in over 200 sampled pregnancies [45].

Irrespective of the route of insertion, continuous ultrasound guidance of the sampling apparatus is a factor of primary importance for the success and safety of CVS. This is reflected in the high rate of fetal loss, which has not been avoided - even in experienced centers - when ultrasound support was poor [39]. Sector scanners give an excellent view of the whole pelvis, and ultrasound guidance of transcervical devices throughout the procedure is very detailed. However, as long as the patient has a full bladder, linear array scanners do as well as sector scanners.

There is general agreement that the optimum time for CVS is from the 9th to the 11th week of gestation, and that the majority of fetal losses occur when the procedure is carried out later (11-13 weeks). The reason for this narrow margin is that before the 8th week the chorion frondosum covers the sac uniformly and CVS is difficult, while after the 11th week the gestation sac covers the uterine cavity, the fetal membranes are more vulnerable, and the placenta becomes very vascular, in such a way that any injury may cause substantial bleeding. Blood loss at the time of biopsy does not appear to correlate with the frequency of miscarriages, although the latter clearly increases with the number of attempts.

The risk of ABO-Rhesus (Rh) isoimmunization following CVS is not negligible since Rh antigens can be identified on fetal erythrocytes after the 32nd day of gestation, and the latter may easily enter the maternal circulation during the procedure (between 42nd and 56th day of gestation). This assumption is supported by the observation that the frequency of ABO-Rh isoimmunization in the first trimester of pregnancy is 3% following a spontaneous abortion and approximately 5% following an induced one. Moreover, in a recent study, alpha-fetoprotein (AFP) levels in the maternal blood increased clearly in most women 6h after CVS [48]. This indicates that fetomaternal bleeding may often take place at the placental interface and supports the standard administration of anti-D to all Rh-negativ women after CVS. To avoid fetomaternal hemorrhage, the number of passages of the cannula, biopsy forceps, or needle should be kept to a minimum. In addition, an increase of AFP may indicate other oncoming difficulties.

Among other complications which can be evaluated with more accuracy, the figures for preterm deliveries, premature rupture of membranes, malformations, and maternal complications (preeclampsia, abruptio placentae, and intrauterine growth retardation) fit well within the mean values for the general population [31]. These procedures do not appear to be associated with abruptio placentae.

In any case, more time is needed to establish the frequencies of fetal losses and obstetrical complications following CVS because the large majority of cases have been carried out very recently, and their results - especially those concerning long-term complications - cannot yet be evaluated with accuracy.

Another important question which remains open as yet concerns the effects of CVS on the growth and development of the offspring. These studies require, undoubtedly, a longer follow-up. However, there is convincing evidence available that babies born following CVS have never presented any problems whatsoever [27, 35, 31, 45].

Conclusions

On the basis of the above information, centers setting up the CVS method should consider the following recommendations:

1. CVS must be carried out under ultrasound guidance and between the 8th and 11th week of pregnancy.
2. The sample must be adequate and in good condition in order to allow an accurate fetal diagnosis. Processing of the sample is best carried out under an inverted or dissecting microscope.
3. All diagnostic cases should be followed

carefully throughout pregnancy; the diagnosis must be confirmed in newborns or abortuses.
4. CVS should be performed only by physicians with technical expertise acquired in centers that provide appropriate genetic counseling and offer second-trimester diagnostic facilities.
5. Training in CVS requires experience on at least 50–100 first-trimester voluntary termination cases before the procedure is attempted on continuing pregnancies. Expertise can be maintained with 100–200 cases annually.

Without doubt, prenatal diagnosis in the first trimester of pregnancy holds a valuable position in clinical obstetrics and genetics. Whether and the extent to which this technique will be established and replace midtrimester amniocentesis and fetoscopy will depend on unanswered questions concerning attitudes toward the safety of sampling procedures and the accuracy of laboratory methods.

References

1. NICHD. National Registry for Amniocentesis Study Group (1976) Midtrimester amniocentesis for prenatal diagnosis. Safety and accuracy. J A M A 236: 1471–1476
2. Report of the Medical Research Council by their Working Party on Amniocentesis (1978) J Obstet Gynaecol 85 (Suppl 2): 1–41
3. Alter BP (1984) Advances in the prenatal diagnosis of hematologic diseases. Blood 64: 329–340
4. Fairweather DVI, Model B, Verdoukas V, Later B, Nathan D, Loukopoulos D, Wood W, Clegg JB, Weatherall D (1978) Antenatal diagnosis of thalassemia major. Br Med J 1: 350
5. Old JM, Ward RHT, Karagözlü F, Petrou M, Modell B, Weatherall D (1982) First trimester fetal diagnosis for hemogobinopathies. Lancet ii: 1416–1417
6. Williamson R, Eskdale J, Coleman DV, Niazi M, Loeffler FE, Modell B (1983) Direct gene analysis of chorionic villi: a possible technique for first trimester antenatal diagnosis of hemoglobinopathies. Lancet ii: 1125–1127
7. Valencti C (1972) Endoamnioscopy and fetal biopsy. A new technique. Am J Obstet Gynecol 114: 561
8. Valencti C (1973) Antenatal detection of hemoglobinopathies. Am J Obstet Gynecol 115: 851
9. Hobbins JC and Mahoney MJ (1974) In utero diagnosis of hemoglobinopathies. N Engl J Med 290: 1065
10. Patrick JE, Perry TB, Kunch RAH (1974) Fetoscopy and fetal blood samgling. A percutaneous approach. AM J Obstet Gynecol 119: 539
11. Antsaklis A, Benzie R, Hughes R (1985) Fetoscopy: fetal visualization and blood sampling in prenatal diagnosis. Marcel Dekker, New York, pp 109–137
12. Proc. Eight annual meeting of the international fetoscopy group. Rotterdam, 1986
13. Loukopoulos D, Karababa P, Antsaklis A, Panourgias J, Boussiou M, Karayannopoulos K, Politis J, Roumbou D, Tassiopoulou A, Fessas P (1986) Prenatal diagnosis of thalassemia and Hb S syndromes in Greece: an evaluation of 1500 cases. Ann NY Acad Sci 445: 357–375
14. Antsaklis A (1981) Fetoscopy at first department of obstetrics and gynaecology, Athens university. In: Rocker I, Laurence KM (eds). Elsevier/North-Holland Biomedical, Amsterdam pp 277–285
15. Prescott T (1976) Needlescope. A transabdominal fetoscope. In: Intrauterine fetal visualization. Excerpta Medica, Amsterdam, p 256
16. Rodeck CH, Campell S (1978) Sampling pure fetal blood by fetoscopy in second trimester of pregnancy. Br Med J II: 728–730
17. Rodeck CH, Campell S (1979) Umbilical cord insertion as a source of pure fetal blood for prenatal diagnosis. Lancet i: 1244–1245
18. Mackenzie IZ, MacLean DA (1980) Pure fetal blood from umbilical cord obtained at fetoscopy. Experience of 125 consecutive cases. Am J Obstet Gynecol 138: 1214–1218
19. Benzie RJ, Pirani BBK (1977) Fetoscopy and anterior placentas. N Engl J Med 296: 573
20. Rodeck CH, Wass D (1981) Sampling pure fetal blood in twin pregnancies by fetoscopy using a single uterine puncture. Prenat Diagn 1: 43–49
21. Antsaklis A, Papantoniou N, Loukopoulos D, Kaskarelis D (1983): Prenatal hemoglobinopathies in twin pregnancies by double simultaneous fetoscopy. Prenat Diagn 31: 21–27
22. Kan YW, Valenti C, Guidotti R, Pieder R (1974) Fetal blood sampling in utero. Lancet i: 80
23. Fairweather DVI, Ward RHT, Model B 1980 Obstetric aspects of mid-trimester fetal blood sampling by needling or fetoscopy. Br J Obstet Gynaecol 87: 87–91
24. Daffos F, Capella-Pavlovsky M, Forestier F (1983) A new procedure for pure fetal blood sampling in utero. Prenat Diagn 3: 271–277
25. Modell B, Ward RHT, Fairweather DVI (1980) Effect of introducing antenatal diagnosis on

reproductive behaviour of families at risk for thalassemia major. Br Med J 1: 1347
26. Blumberg BO, Globus MS, Hanson KH (1975) The psychological sequelae of abortion performed for genetic indication. Am J Obstet Gynecol 122: 799–808
27. Goosens M, Dumez Y, Kaplan L, Lupker M, Chabret C, Henrion R, Rosa J (1983) Prenatal diagnosis of sickle cell anemia in the first trimester of pregnancy. N Engl J Med 309: 833
28. Elles RG, Williamson R, Niazi M, Coleman DV, Horwell D (1983) Absence of maternal contamination of chorionic villi used for fetal-gene analysis. N Engl J Med 308: 1433
29. Pirastu M, Doherthy M, Galanello R, Cao A, Kau YM (1986) Frequent crossing over in human DNA generates multiple chromosomes contraining the sickle and β-thalassemia genes and increases HbF production. Blood 6 (Suppl): 75a (Abstr), 19
30. Orkin SH, Markham AF, Kazazian HH Jr (1983) Direct detection of the common Mediterranean β-thalassemia gene with synthetic DNA probes an alternative approach for prenatal diagnosis. J Clin Invest 71: 775
31. Brambati B, Ordini A, Ferrazzi E, Lazani A (1985) Chorionic villi sampling: general methodological and clinical approach. In: Fraccaro M, Simoni G, Brambati B (eds.) First trimester fetal diagnosis. Springer, Berlin Heidelerg New York, pp 7–18
32. Hogge WA, Shouberg SA, Golbus MS (1986) Chorionic villi sampling. Experience of the first 1000 cases. Am J Ostet Gynecol 154: 1249–1252
33. Simoni G, Brambati B, Danesino C, Terzoli GL, Romitti L. Rossella F, Fraccaro M (1984) Diagnostic application of first trimester trophoplast sampling in 100 pregnancies. Hum Genet 66: 252–259
34. Antsaklis A (1987) First trimester prenatal diagnosis chorionic villi sampling (CVS). In: Loukopoulos (ed) Prenatal diagnosis of thalassemia. Editor: Loukopoulos D, CRC Press Boca Raton, Inc USA
35. Kazy Z, Razovsky IS, Bakharev VA (1982). Chorionic biopsy in early pregnancy. A method of early prenatal diagnosis for inherited disorders. Prenat Diagn 2: 2
36. Ginsberg N, Brandt T, Cadkin A, Verlinsky Y, Pergament E (1985) Technical aspects of chorionic villi sampling in first trimester fetal diagnosis. In: Fraccaro M, Simoni G, Brambatti B (eds). First trimester fetal diagnosis. Springer Springer, Berlin, Heidelberg, New York, p 25
37. Ward RHT, Model B, Petrou M, Karagozlu F, Douratsos E (1983). A method of chorionic villus sampling in the first trimester of pregnancy under real time ultrasonic guidance. Br Med J 2: 1542
38. Brambati B, Simoni G (1983) Diagnosis of fetal trisomy 21 in first trimester. Lancet i: 586
39. Ward RHT, Model B, Petrou M, Kanakpougsukdi S, Penketh RC (1985) Chorionic villi sampling in a high risk population using the Portex cannula. In: Fraccaro M, Simoni G, Brambati B (eds.) First trimester fetal diagnosis. Springer, Berlin Heidelberg New York p 38
40. Dumez Y, Goossens M, Bone J, Poenaru L, Dommergues M, Henrion R (1985) Chorionic villi sampling using a rigid forceps under ultrasound control. In: Fraccaro M, Simoni G, Brambati B, (eds.) First trimester fetal diagnosis. Springer, Berlin Heidelberg New York p 38
41. Smidt-Jensen S, Hahnemann N, Jensen PKA, Therkelsen AJ (1984) Experience with transabdominal fine needle biopsy from chorionic villi in the first trimester: an alternative to amniocentesis. Clin Genet 26: 272
42. Maxwell D, Czepulkowski B, Lipford R, Heaton D, Coleman D (1986) Transabdominal chorionic villi sampling. Lencet i: 123–126
43. Holzgreve W, Miny P (1985) Improved echogenicity of the catheter for chorion villi sampling. In: Fraccaro M, Simoni G, Brambati B (eds) First trimester fetal diagnosis. Springer, Berlin Heidelberg New York, p 63
44. Jackson LG, Wapner RJ, Grebner EE, Barr MA (1985) Fetal genetic diagnosis by chorionic villus sampling. In: Filkins K, Russo J (eds) Human prenatal diagnosis. Mercel-Deccer, New York p 285
45. Jackson LG (1986) Chorinic villi sampling. Latest news, newsletter 18, Sept 1986
46. Elias S, Simpson JL, Martin AO, Sabbagh R, Bombard A, Rosinsky BJ, Baum LD (1986) Chorionic villus sampling in continuing pregnancies. Am J Obstet Gynecol 154:1349-1352
47. Tietung hospital, Department of obstetrics and gynecology. Fetal prediction by sex chromatin of chorionic villi cells during early pregnancy. Clin Med J 1: 117
48. Ward RHT, Grudzinskas JC, Bolton AE, Modell B, Kanakpousukdi S, Petrou M, Chard T (1985) Fetoplacental products as a prognostic guide following chorionic villi sampling. In: Fraccaso M, Simoni G, Brambati B (eds) First trimester fetal giagnosis. Springer, Berlin Heidelberg New York, p 74

Subject Index

MIX
Papier aus verantwortungsvollen Quellen
Paper from responsible sources
FSC® C105338

If you have any concerns about our products,
you can contact us on
ProductSafety@springernature.com

In case Publisher is established outside the EU,
the EU authorized representative is:
Springer Nature Customer Service Center GmbH
Europaplatz 3, 69115 Heidelberg, Germany

Printed by Libri Plureos GmbH
in Hamburg, Germany